101
INSPIRING
LIVES

Tanvir Khan

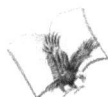

V&S PUBLISHERS

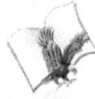

Published by:

V&S PUBLISHERS

F-2/16, Ansari road, Daryaganj, New Delhi-110002
☎ 23240026, 23240027 • *Fax:* 011-23240028
Email: info@vspublishers.com • *Website:* www.vspublishers.com

Regional Office : Hyderabad
5-1-707/1, Brij Bhawan (Beside Central Bank of India Lane)
Bank Street, Koti, Hyderabad - 500 095
☎ 040-24737290
E-mail: vspublishershyd@gmail.com

Branch Office : Mumbai
Jaywant Industrial Estate, 1st Floor–108, Tardeo Road
Opposite Sobo Central Mall, Mumbai – 400 034
☎ 022-23510736
E-mail: vspublishersmum@gmail.com

Follow us on:

DISCLAIMER

Printed at Repro Knowledgecast Limited, Thane

Publisher's Note————————————————

In keeping with the philosophy of bringing out books of immortal values, V&S Publishers has brought out this book, *101 Inspiring Lives*. This information-packed book chronicles the lives of 101 of the most influential personalities whose achievements have helped shape the modern world.

The list includes famous statesmen and women, entrepreneurs, scientists, social reformers, film artists, sportsmen and women, among others. Also included in the book are eminent people that include those who have achieved distinction as writers, musicians, business persons, philanthropists, etc.

The selection has been made out of personalities from several countries across the globe. Enjoy reading about Mahatma Gandhi, Jawaharlal Nehru, Abraham Lincoln, John Kennedy, Albert Einstein, JRD Tata, Lata Mangeshkar, Pele, Sachin Tendulkar, etc. These famous personalities have influenced our lives, and have become a source of constant inspiration and motivation for all of us.

The text is organised category-wise for easy access and reference.

Each biography includes a *trivia,* a *quote,* the successes, failures and awards associated with these great people to inspire the readers and satisfy their curious instincts.

So read on the success stories of each of these great personalities and discover for yourself if you can imbibe their traits during your growing years to make it big in your life.

Contents

ACTORS/DIRECTORS

ARTISTS

BUSINESSMEN/ENTREPRENEURS

HISTORIANS/HISTORIC FIGURES

SINGERS/MUSICIANS

POLITICIANS/DIPLOMATS

SCIENTISTS/INVENTORS

SOCIAL REFORMERS

SPORTSPERSONS

WRITERS/POETS/LYRICISTS

ACTORS/ DIRECTORS

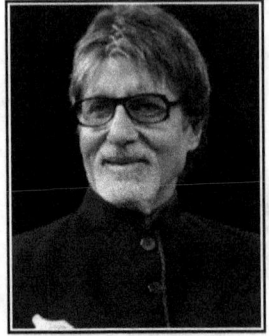

AMITABH BACHCHAN

Born on October 11, 1942 to well-known poet Harivansh Rai Bachchan and Teji Bachchan, Amitabh Bachchan is a famous Bollywood actor since 1969.

Known as the 'Angry Young Man' of Bollywood, he is popularly called Big B or Amitji. After studying at the Boys' High School, he took up arts as his subject in Sherwood College.

Amitabh Bachchan started his film career as a voice narrator in *Bhuvan Shome* in 1969. He got his first opportunity as an actor in *Saat Hindustani.*

Having starred in many films including *Parwaana, Reshma Aur Shera, Guddi* and many others during 1969-1972, he married Jaya Bhaduri after his first hit film, *Zanjeer* in 1973. The couple has a son and a daughter. His son, Abhishek Bachchan is also a popular Bollywood star.

The year 1975 had been a year of blockbuster hits for him, in which he gave films like *Deewar* and *Sholay.*

Some of the other films to his credit are *Amar Akbar Anthony, Kabhie Kabhie, Muqaddar Ka Sikandar, Trishul, Ram Balram, Mr. Natwarlal, Dostana, Silsila, Shaan, Lawaaris* and *Shakti.*

After an injury on the sets of a film, he had decided to quit films and enter politics but returned to films again in 988 with *Shahenshah.*

He is conferred with **Padma Shri** in 1984 and **Padma Bhushan** in 2001. Having more than 100 films to his name, Amitabh Bachchan is still going strong.

In addition to acting, Bachchan or the Big B has also worked as a playback singer, a film producer and a television presenter in one of the most popular T.V. shows, *Kaun Banega Crorepati.* He was also an elected member of the Indian Parliament from 1984 to 1987.

Trivia

He was initially named *Inquilab* by his father, but later changed to his current name on the advice of a friend.

CHARLIE CHAPLIN

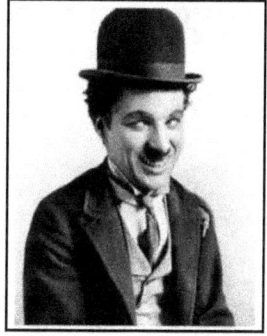

Born on April 16, 1889, in London to Charles and Hannah Chaplin, Sir Charles Spencer Chaplin was a British comedian, producer, writer, director and composer.

He is best known for his work during the silent film era. Famous for his *Little Tramp* character, the sweet little man with a bowler hat, moustache and cane, Chaplin was one of film's first superstars, elevating in a way one could have ever imagined.

Charlie Chaplin's rise was a true 'rags-to-riches' story. His father abandoned Chaplin, his mother and his brother, Sydney.

Chaplin began his official acting career at the age of eight, touring with The Eight Lancashire Lads. At 18, he began touring with Fred Karno's vaudeville troupe, joining them on the troupe's 1910 US tour.

After having made many films, Charlie Chaplin, Douglas Fairbanks, Mary Pickford and DW Griffith formed the United Artists (A) in 1919.

He became the most famous film star before the end of World War I. Chaplin used slapstick, mime and other visual comedy routines and continued well into the era of the talkies, though his films decreased from the end of the 1920s.

Chaplin's life and career was full of scandals and controversy. Amid those controversies, Chaplin has seen a good career. Chaplin died of natural causes on December 25, 1977 at his home in Switzerland.

Trivia

Chaplin married four times and had a total of 11 children. In 1918, he married Mildred Harris. The couple had a son who just lived for three days. After their divorce in 1920, he married Lita Grey in 1924. The couple had two children. Then, he married Paulette Goddard in 1936 and his final marriage was to Oona O'Neill in 1943. Oona gave birth to eight children.

ELIZABETH TAYLOR

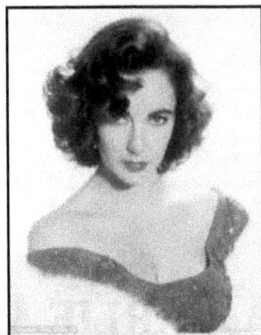

Born on February 27, 1932, Dame Elizabeth Rosemond 'Liz' Taylor was a British-American actress. As a child star with the Metro-Goldwyn-Mayer (MGM), she became a great screen actress of Hollywood's Golden Age.

Elizabeth lived in London until the age of seven, after which the family left for the United States when clouds of war began brewing in Europe in 1939.

Taylor was known for her acting ability, glamorous lifestyle, beauty and distinctive violet eyes. Her first venture on the screen was in *There's One Born Every Minute* in 1942. It was released when she was ten years old. Later, Elizabeth was picked up by the MGM.

She did many films with the studio, the first one being *Lassie Come Home* in 1943. She had minuscule parts in her next two films – *The White Cliffs of Dover* and *Jane Eyre*.

She gained widespread popularity with MGM's *National Velvet* in 1944. In 1947, she starred in *Life with Father* with popular actors like William Powell, Irene Dunne and Zasu Pitts.

Her busiest year was 1954, with roles in *Rhapsody, Beau Brummell, The Last Time I Saw Paris* and *Elephant Walk*. Some of her other successful films include *Raintree County, Cat on a Hot Tin Roof, Suddenly* and *Last Summer*. She also won an **Oscar** for *Butterfield 8*.

Taylor died of congestive heart failure in March 2011 at the age of 79, having suffered many years of ill health.

Trivia

She married eight times in her lifetime and has four children.

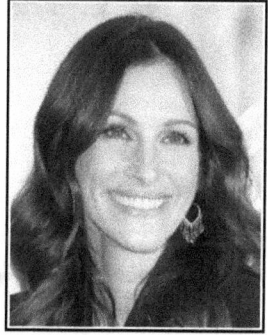

JULIA ROBERTS

Born in Smyrna, Georgia on October 28, 1967, Julia Fiona Roberts had never dreamt that she would become the most popular actress in America. As a child, due to her love of animals, Julia originally wanted to be a veterinarian but later studied journalism.

After her brother Eric Roberts achieved some success in Hollywood, Julia decided to try acting. Her first break came in 1988 youth-oriented movies, *Mystic Pizza* and *Satisfaction*. The movies introduced her to a new audience who instantly fell in love with this pretty woman.

Julia's biggest success was in the signature movie, *Pretty Woman*, for which Julia got an **Oscar nomination** and also won the **People's Choice Award** for Favourite Actress.

Audience would always love Julia best in romantic comedies. With *My Best Friend's Wedding* in 1997, Julia gave the genre fresh life that had been lacking in Hollywood for some time.

Off screen, after a brief marriage, Julia has been linked with several other actors. Julia also got involved with UNICEF charities and has made visits to many different countries, including Haiti and India in order to promote goodwill. Julia is one of the most popular and sought-after talents in Hollywood.

Trivia

She was chosen one of the '50 Most Beautiful People in the World' by the People magazine in 2000.

Quote

"Happiness isn't happiness unless there's a violin-playing goat."

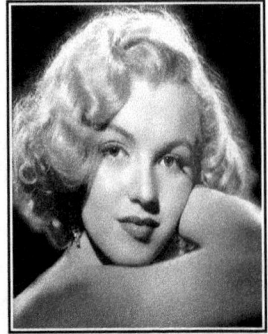

MARILYN MONROE

Marilyn Monroe was born as Norma Jeane Mortenson on June 1, 1926, in Los Angeles General Hospital. Prior to her birth, Marilyn's father headed north to San Francisco, abandoning the family in Los Angeles. Marilyn grew up not knowing for sure who her father really was. Her mother, Gladys, had entered into several relationships, further confusing her daughter as to who it was who fathered her.

Her first film was in 1947 with a bit part in *The Shocking Miss Pilgrim*. Her next production was not much better, a bit in the eminently forgettable *Scudda Hoo! Scudda Hay!* (1948). Two of the three brief scenes she appeared wound up on the cutting room floo . Later, she was given a somewhat better role as waitress, Evie in *Dangerous Years*. However, Fox declined to renew her contract, so she went back to modelling and the acting school.

Columbia gave her a six-month contract in the B movie, *Ladies of the Chorus* (1948) in which she sang two numbers. Joseph L. Mankiewiez saw her in a small part in *The Asphalt Jungle* (1950) and put her in *All About Eve* (1950), resulting in resigning her to a seven-year contract with the *20th Century Fox Film Corporation*. *Niagara* (1953) and *Gentlemen Prefer Blondes* (1953) launched her as a sex symbol superstar.

The work on her last picture, *The Misfit* (1961), written for her by departing husband Miller was interrupted by exhaustion. She was dropped from the unfinished *Something's Got to Give* (1962) due to chronic lateness and drug dependency. Four months later, she was found dead in her Brentwood home of a drug overdose, adjudged "probable suicide".

Trivia
She has voted the 'Sexiest Woman of the Century' by the People magazine. [1999]

Quote
"A career is wonderful, but you can't curl up with it on a cold night."

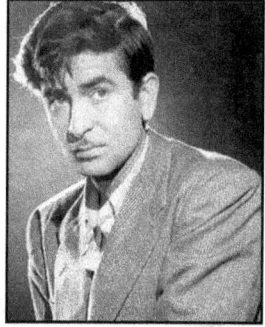

RAJ KAPOOR

A legendary actor, director, and producer of many Bollywood movies, Raj Kapoor was born on December 14, 1924 at Peshawar in the North-West Frontier Province of what is now Pakistan.

Raj Kapoor began his career as a clapper boy assisting director Kidar Sharma. He appeared in films for the first time in the film *Inquilab* in 1935 at the age of eleven.

The big break came to him when he played the main lead in *Neel Kamal* in 1947. He established his studio, **RK Films,** when he was 24 and became the youngest director of his era in the Hindi cinema.

His directorial debut in *Aag* was a thumping success. He directed many films that are still remembered and loved – *Barsaat* (1949), *Awaara* (1951), *Shri 420* (1955), and *Sangam* (1964). He also starred in a number of the films, he directed, often with his real-life love interest, actress, Nargis.

Films like *Mera Naam Joker, Bobby, Satyam Shivam Sundaram* and *Ram Teri Ganga Maili* are also to his credit.

At the age of 22, in 1946, Raj Kapoor was married to Krishna Malhotra in a traditional family-arranged wedding. The couple have five children – Randhir, Ritu, Rishi, Rima and Rajiv.

Raj Kapoor suffered from asthma in his later years and died of complications in 1988. He was working on the movie *Henna* when he died. The film was later completed by his son, Randhir Kapoo .

Noted film personalities of the present Bollywood, Karisma and Kareena Kapoor are the granddaughters of Raj and Krishna Kapoor, being the daughters of their eldest son, Randhir by his wife Babita. His younger brothers Shammi Kapoor and Shashi Kapoor were also actors. Rishi Kapoor, the younger son of Raj Kapoor, too is a great actor.

Trivia

Raj Kapoor's performance in Awaara, was ranked one of the "Top-Ten Performances of all time", by the Time magazine of the Indian Cinema.

SHAHRUKH KHAN

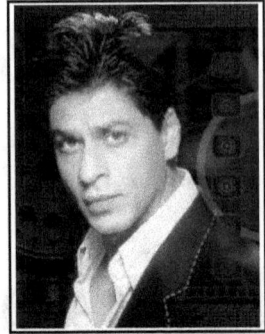

Shahrukh Khan was born on November 2, 1965. Shahrukh started his career with a TV serial called *Fauji* in 1988 that won him instant recognition. He has also acted in another TV soap called 'Circus' in 1989.

Being equally brilliant in studies and sports, he completed his education from Delhi. He fell in love with Gauri Chibba, and after many objections from her parents, married her before he got his break in Bollywood. The couple has two children.

Often referred to as 'the King of Bollywood', Shahrukh has acted in over 70 Hindi films

He made his film debut in *Deewana* in 1992. The Government of India honoured him with the **Padma Shri** for his contributions towards the Indian Cinema in 2005.

Since 1992, he has been part of numerous commercial successes as well as has delivered a variety of critically acclaimed performances.

Some of his successful films include *Dilwale Dulhaniya Le Jayenge* (1995), *Kuch Kuch Hota Hai* (1998), *Kabhi Khushi Kabhie Gham* (2001), *Kal Ho Naa Ho* (2003), *Veer-Zaara* (2004), *Kabhi Alvida Naa Kehna* (2006), *Chak De! India* (2007), *Om Shanti Om* (2007), *Rab Ne Bana Di Jodi* (2008), *My Name Is Khan* (2010).

Shahrukh also branched out into film production and television presenting. He is the co-owner of two production companies, Dreamz Unlimited and Red Chillies Entertainment. Shahrukh is also the owner of the IPL cricket team, 'Kolkata Knight Riders'.

Shahrukh and his wife, Gauri Khan, own the production company "Red Chillies Entertainments" which Shahrukh started for his friend and colleague – Farah Khan, director/choreographer, for her debut directorial film – *Main Hoon Na* (2004).

Trivia

Khan has won fourteen Filmfare Awards for his work in Indian films and out of which, eight are in the Best Actor category (a record).

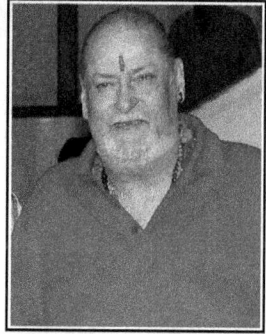

Shammi Kapoor

Born on October 21, 1931, Shammi Kapoor was a famous Indian actor and director. Shamsher Raj or 'Shammi' Kapoor, son of actor Prithviraj Kapoor and Ramsarni 'Rama' Mehra Kapoor, moved into filmmaking with his father's company, Prithvi Theatres.

He started his career in 1953, but his movies did not succeed at the box office. He worked in films like *Coffee House* and *Rangin Raaten* from 1955 to 1957 but could not make his name.

His film *Tumsa Nahin Dekha* in 1957 was a turning point in his career. The new look with short hair and no moustache created a different persona, all together. The film was followed with many more hits like *Junglee, Teesri Manzil, Brahmachari* and many more.

He had married actress Geeta Bali in 1955. She died of smallpox in 1965. Shammi Kapoor married again to Queen of Bhavanagar Neila Devi in 1969.

Andaz was his last film as a leading actor in 1971. However, he continued to do supporting roles in several films in later years. He also directed two films, *Manoranjan* and *Bundal Baaz.* Later, Shammi founded the *Internet Users Community of India,* where he used to speak directly to his fans and made online videos.

Many of his family members including his elder brother, Raj Kapoor and younger brother, Shashi Kapoor, their spouses, grandchildren, are or have been into the film industr .

His last film was *Rockstar* with his great-nephew, Ranbir Kapoor. Shammi Kapoor died on August 14, 2011 due to chronic renal failure.

Trivia

Shammi Kapoor was one of the first persons in India to contribute in the field of Internet. Shammi Kapoor has two children, Aditya Raj and Kanchan, both from his previous wife.

ARTISTS

Leonardo Da Vinci

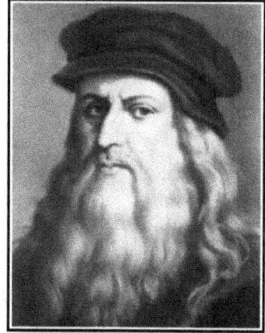

Most people are known for mastering a specific field. But, such is not the case with Leonardo Da Vinci. He was a curious soul. His curiosity led him to explore everything that he came across. As a result, he was an expert in many fields unlike anyone before or after him

Leonardo was born on April 15, 1452 in Anchiano, Republic of Florence (now in Italy). His father was a landlord and mother was a peasant woman.

Gradually recognising Leonardo's hidden artistic talent, his father introduced him to the renowned artist, Andrea del Verrocchio. Leonardo received training of painting, sculpting and mechanical arts. He got admitted into the painters' guild of Florence in 1472 as his artistic abilities flourished

He continued learning at the workshop for five years after which he worked independently. He died on May 2, 1519 in Cloux, France.

Leonardo is known for his famous paintings – *The Last Supper*, *The Mona Lisa* and *The Vitruvian Man: The Proportions of the Human Figure*.

Besides being known as a painter, he is known as a sculptor, an architect, a scientist and an engineer. To name a few, he had also explored areas like Anatomy, Geology, Botany and Archaeology.

He had explained the fundamental theory of evolution, hundreds of years before Darwin and also of a flying machine. Many inventions and discoveries made after him seem to have been drawn from such fundamental theories of Leonardo.

Trivia

Leonardo da Vinci's famous painting, The Mona Lisa is of Lisa del Giocondo, the wife of a silk merchant. The husband had hired Leonardo to paint his wife's portrait. Today it is displayed in the Louvre Museum in Paris.

Quote

"Art is never finished, only abandoned."

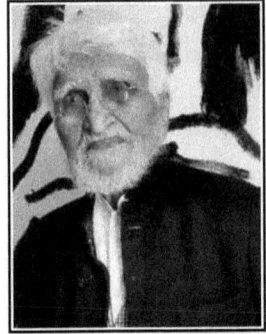

M.F. HUSSAIN

Popularly known as the 'Picasso of India', celebrated painter Maqbool Fida Hussain earned both fame and wrath for his paintings. M.F. Hussain, who died in June 2011, was an accomplished painter mostly famous for his paintings on Indian women.

At the age of 20, he moved to Mumbai determined to become an artist. He started his career in 1937 by painting *cinema hoardings* to earn his livelihood. Hussain's painting, 'Sunhera Sansaar' in an annual exhibition of the Bombay Art Society in 1947 marked his entry as a known artist.

He became a popular artist through a series of his exhibitions since 1948. He organised his first solo exhibition in 1952 and then there was no looking back for him.

He attracted a lot of controversies for his nude paintings of Hindu gods and goddesses. He was arrested and charged with hurting sentiments of the people. Organisations like 'Shiv Sena' and 'Vishwa Hindu Parishad' opposed such paintings. Following his arrest, the court had ordered that an artist has freedom of expression but within the limit of not hurting the sentiments of people.

One of Hussain's films, *Meenaxi: A Tale of Three Cities* was also pulled out of theatres after some Muslim organisations claimed that one of the songs in the film contained words directly taken from the Quran

His first film, *Through the Eyes of a Painter,* made in 1967 received recognition at the Berlin Film Festival.

M.F. Hussain was conferred with respectable awards like the **Padma Shri, Padma Bhushan** and **Padma Vibhushan**.

Trivia

Born in Pandharpur of Madhya Pradesh on September 17, 1915, M.F. Hussain got married to Fazila in 1941 and had two daughters, Raisa and Aqueela and three sons, Mustafa, Shamshad and Owais. His single canvases have fetched up about 2 million dollars.

MICHELANGELO BUONARROTI

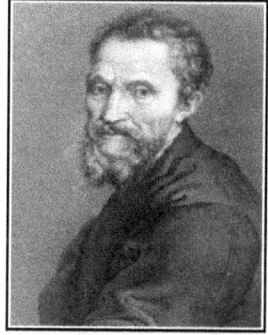

Michelangelo Buonarroti was born on March 6, 1475 in Italy in a middle-class family. His father enjoyed a reputed position in the government and hence considered his son's desire to be an artist as disgraceful.

Earlier, Michelangelo started to learn grammar but hated it. He started working as an apprentice under painter Domenico Ghirlandaio in Florence at the age of thirteen.

During his apprenticeship, he got access to the antique collection of Lorenzo de' Medici. This acquaintance gave Michelangelo the opportunity to meet great scientist and even trained by Bertoldo di Giovanni, the resident sculptor of the Medici family. This arrangement enhanced the artistic skill possessed by Michelangelo.

His major works were mostly left unfinished on account of their scale. Pope Julius II assigned him the task to build his tomb, which was to include 40 life-size statues in 1505. The project took 40 long years of Michelangelo's life.

The Pope gave him another project in 1508 which was to paint the ceiling of the Sistine Chapel. He painted stories from Genesis on the ceiling, unlike using the traditional technique of painting a single figure. After completing the ceiling, he continued his work on the Pope's tomb.

However, the project came to a stop when Julius died in 1513. Three years later, he was commissioned to paint the back wall of the *Sistine Chapel with The Last Judgement*. In 1555, he started working on *Pieta* in St. Peter's church, Milan, during which he fell ill and passed away in 1564.

Trivia
Michelangelo built an 18 feet tall statue of David in Florence in 1501.

🎥 🎥

NICHOLAS ROERICH

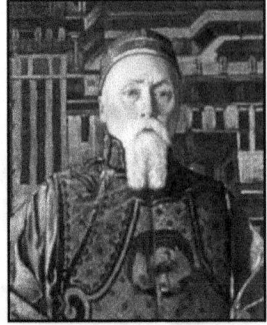

A lso known as Nikolai Konstantinovich Rerikh, Nicholas Roerich (September 27, 1874 to December 13, 1947), was a Russian mystic, painter, philosopher, scientist, writer, traveller and public figure.

From childhood, Nicholas Roerich was attracted to painting, archaeology, history and the abundant cultural heritage of the East.

He was a prolific artist. He created thousands of paintings and about 30 literary works. Many of his paintings are exhibited in well-known museums of the world.

Roerich was also an author and a founder of an international movement for the defence of culture. He was also the initiator of an international pact for the protection of artistic and academic institutions and historical sites called the 'Roerich's Pact'.

Roerich earned several nominations for the **Nobel Prize**.

Members of Roerich's family occupied prominent military and administrative posts in Russia since the reign of Peter I. Nicholas Roerich's father, Konstantin Fedorovich was a well-known notary, who was born in Courland.

Roerich's mother, Maria Vasil'evna Kalashnikova was descended from a long line of merchants and traders. Among the friends of the Roerich's family, were famous personalities, such as D Mendeleyev, N Kostomarov, M Mikeshin, L Ivanovsky and many others.

Trivia

Roerich in translation from the ancient Scandinavian means 'rich of fame'.

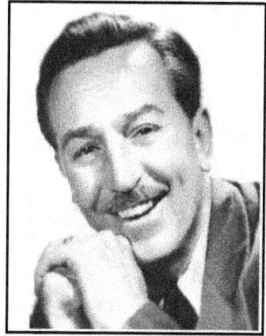

WALT DISNEY

Walt Disney was born on December 5, 1901 in Chicago Illinois. His father, Elias Disney and mother, Flora Call Disney had five children, four boys and a girl. His father, a strict and religious man, who often physically abused his children, was working as a building contractor when Walter was born.

Walt had very early interests in art. He used to sell his drawings to neighbours and make extra money. He pursued his arts, by studying art and photography at McKinley High School in Chicago. He had grown his love for nature and wildlife and family and community, which were a large part of agrarian living. Walt was encouraged by his mother and elder brother, Roy to pursue his talents.

On returning from France, he opened his own company which fell bankrupt and then, with twenty dollars in his hand, he headed towards Hollywood. Walt became a recognised Hollywood figure after making success of his 'Alice Comedies'. In 1925, he married Lillian Bounds, in Lewiston. Later on they were blessed with two daughters, Diane and Sharon.

And then his productions fetched him many awards till 1937. During the next five years, **Walt Disney Studios** completed other full-length animated classics, such as *Pinocchio, Fantasia, Dumbo* and *Bambi*.

Walt Disney's dream of a clean and organised amusement park, came true, as **Disneyland Park** opened in 1955.

Trivia

During the fall of 1918, Disney attempted to enlist for military service but got rejected because of being underage. Instead, he joined the Red Cross and spent a year driving an ambulance and chauffeuring Red Cross officials in France. His ambulance was covered with Disney cartoons.

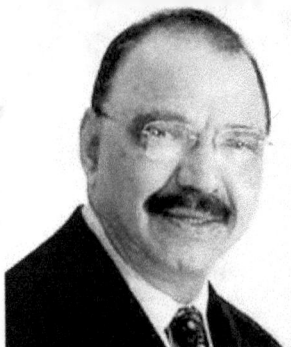

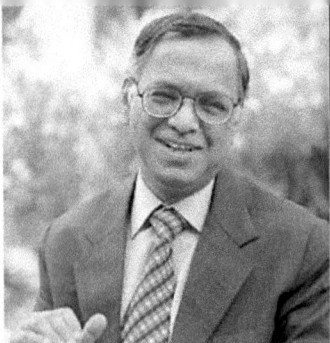

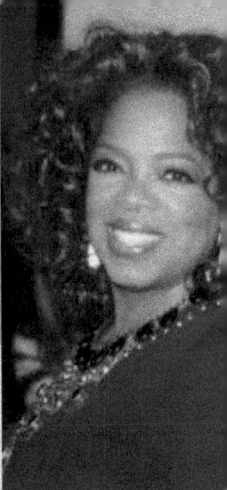

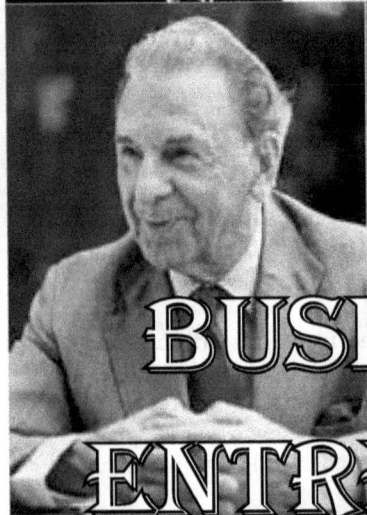

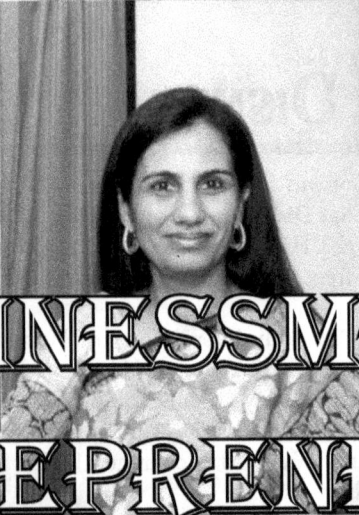

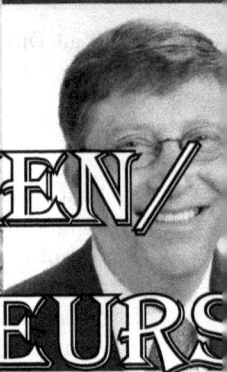

BUSINESSMEN/ENTREPRENEURS

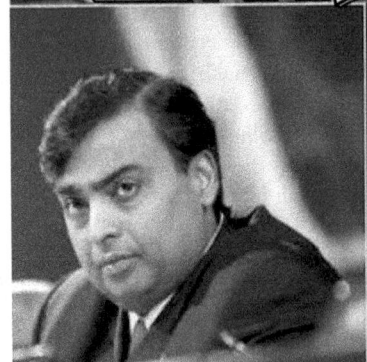

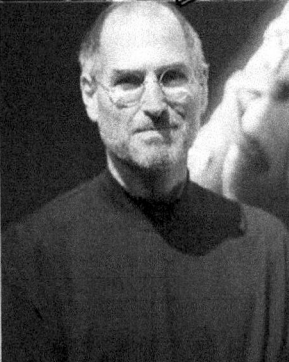

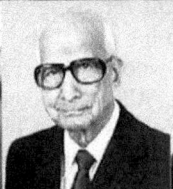

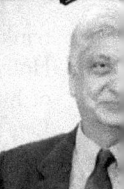

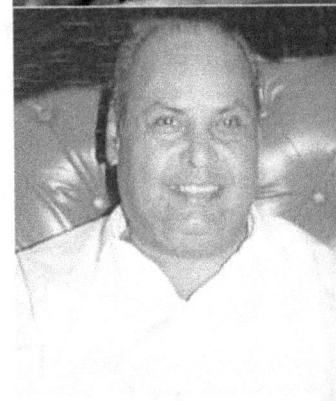

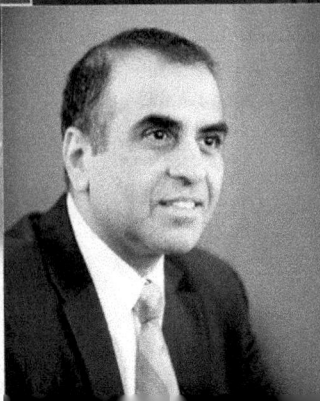

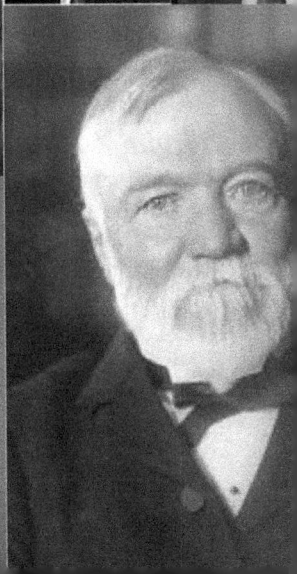

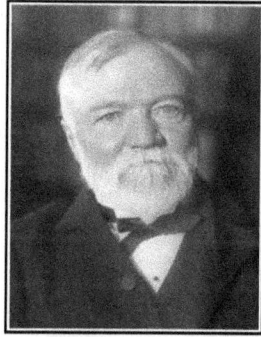

ANDREW CARNEGIE

Andrew Carnegie, (November 25, 1835 – August 11, 1919) was a Scottish-American businessman, entrepreneur and philanthropist. He led the enormous expansion of the American steel industry in the late 19th century.

Carnegie was born in Scotland and migrated to the United States. He started working as a factory worker in a bobbin factory. Later, he became a bill logger for the owner of the company and then a messenger boy. Progressing up the ranks of a telegraph company, he built the Pittsburgh's Carnegie Steel Company, which was later merged with Elbert H Gary's Federal Steel Company. It further merged with several smaller companies to create the US Steel.

He built the *Carnegie Hall* and later turned to philanthropy and interests in education. He founded the 'Carnegie Corporation of New York', 'Carnegie Endowment for International Peace', 'Carnegie Institution of Washington', 'Carnegie Mellon University' and the 'Carnegie Museums of Pittsburgh'.

Carnegie devoted the remainder of his life to large-scale philanthropy, with special emphasis on local libraries, world peace, education and scientific research.

Trivia

He cemented his name as one of the 'Captains of Industry' after he founded the Carnegie Steel Company. By the 1890s, the company was the largest and most profitable industrial enterprise in the world. Carnegie, later, sold it for $480 million to JP Morgan, who then created the US Steel.

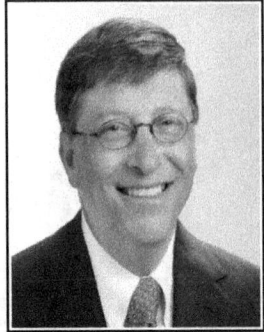

BILL GATES

Born on October 28, 1955 in Seattle, **William Henry 'Bill' Gates III** is an American businessman, philanthropist, author, investor and current Chairman of Microsoft, the software company he founded with **Paul Allen**.

He had an early interest in software and began programming computers at the age of thirteen. Bill Gates became a student at the Harvard University in 1973. His life changed in January 1975 when a magazine carried a cover story on a $350 microcomputer, the Altair, made by a firm called the MITS.

He dropped out of the University and started working as a software designer. Allen and Gates planned to develop software for the newly emerging personal computer market.

The company, **Microsoft** became famous for their computer operating systems and business deals.

Gates proceeded to make a fortune from the licensing of an operating system, MS-DOS that IBM needed for their new personal computer.

On November 10, 1983, Microsoft Corporation was formally announced Microsoft Windows, a next-generation operating system.

Bill Gates married Melinda French Gates in January 1994. The couple has three children.

Besides being the most famous businessman of the late 1990s, Gates has also distinguished himself as a philanthropist.

Bill Gates and his wife Melinda have endowed the Bill and Melinda Gates Foundation with huge amounts of money to support philanthropic initiatives in the areas of global health and learning.

Trivia

The Gates's home is on a hill overlooking Lake Washington in Medina. According to sources in 2006, the total value of the propterty was 125 million dollars.

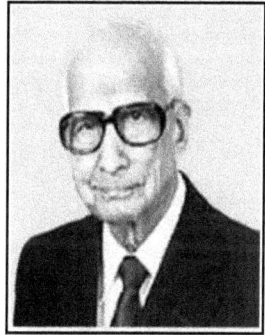

G. D. BIRLA

Ghanshyam Das Birla was born on April 10, 1894. He was an Indian businessman and member of the influential Birla amily.

His grandfather, Shiv Narayan Birla was a traditional Marwari moneylender. Ghanshyam Das Birla entered the business arena during the time of the First World War. He established a cotton mill in Sabzi Mandi, Delhi and later on established the Keshoram Cotton Mills and also the jute business shifting his base to Calcutta (Kolkata), the capital city of Bengal, the world's largest jute producing region.

Ghanshyam Das Birla is considered as a doyen of Indian Industry. He was the founder of the **Federation of Indian Chambers of Commerce and Industry** (FICCI). He is also popularly known as the builder of **Birla Mandirs**. In 1919, the Birla Brothers Limited was formed and a mill was set up in Gwalior. In 1930s, G.D. Birla set up Sugar and Paper mills. In 1940s, he ventured into the territory of cars and established Hindustan Motors. After independence, Ghanshyam Das Birla invested in tea and textiles through a series of acquisitions of erstwhile European companies. He also expanded and diversified into cement, chemicals, rayon and steel tubes.

He was also the founder of various educational institutions. Pilani has today evolved into one of India's best engineering schools. He also established many temples, planetariums and hospitals. Ghanshyam Das Birla died in 1983 at the age of 90. In his honour, the G.D. Birla Award for scientific research has been established to encourage the scientists for their contribution in various fields of scientific research. In 1957, he was awarded India's second highest civilian honour, the **Padma Vibhushan** by the Government of India.

Trivia

There is a memorial to Ghanshyam Das Birla in the Golders Green Crematorium, Hoop Lane, London.

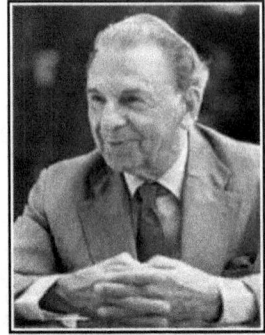

J.R.D. TATA

Jehangir Ratanji Dadabhoy Tata or JRD Tata (July 29, 1904 – November 29, 1993) was a pioneer aviator and important businessman of India.

Born in Paris, Tata was the second child of Ratanji Dadabhoy Tata and Suzanne Brière. His father was the first cousin of Jamsetji Tata, who was a pioneer industrialist in India. He spent much of his childhood in France.

JRD Tata was inspired early by aviation pioneer Louis Blériot and took to flying. On ebruary 10, 1929, Tata got the first pilot licence in India.

Came to be known as the Father of Indian Civil Aviation, Tata founded India's first commercial airline, 'Tata Airlines', in 1932, which came to be known as Air India in 1946.

The assets of the Tata Group grew from US$100 million to over US$5 billion under Tata's chairmanship.

JRD Tata was awarded the **'Bharat Ratna'** in 1992 and the 'Legion of Honour' from the French government in 1954.

Starting with 14 enterprises, Tata & Sons became a conglomerate of 95 enterprises, half a century later in 1988.

Trivia

JRD Tata was famous for succeeding in business while maintaining high ethical standards, refusing to bribe politicians or use the black market.

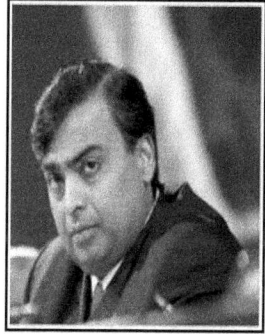

MUKESH AMBANI

Mukesh Ambani is the face of new emerging India. He is the Chairman and Managing Director of Reliance Industries Limited, India's largest private sector company. Born on April 19, 1957 in Mumbai, his father Dhirubhai Ambani was then a small businessman who later on rose to become one of the legends of the Indian industry. Mukesh also owns the Indian Premier League team, 'Mumbai Indians'. He was educated at Abaay Morischa School in Mumbai and completed his graduation with a bachelor's degree in chemical engineering from the UDCT.

Mukesh Ambani joined the Reliance Industries in 1981 and initiated Reliance's backward integration from textiles into polyester fibres and further into petrochemicals. In this process, he directed the creation of 60 new, world-class manufacturing facilities involving diverse technologies that have raised Reliance's manufacturing capacities from less than a million tonnes to twelve million tonnes per year. He has created the world's largest petrol refinery at Jamnagar, Gujarat, India, with a present capacity of 660,000 barrels per day. He was chosen the **businessman of the year, 2007** by a public poll in India conducted by the NDTV. He was ranked 42nd among the World's Most Respected Business Leaders and second among the four Indian CEOs featured in a survey conducted by Pricewaterhouse Coopers. Mukesh Ambani has many achievements and honours to his name. He was chosen as the ET Business Leader of the Year 2006 and was ranked 42nd among the World's Most Respected Business Leaders. He was conferred the World Communication Award for the Most Influential Person in Telecommunications in 2004 by Total Telecom.

Trivia

Mukesh got enrolled for an MBA from the Stanford University, but completed only one year of the two-year program.

NAGAVARA RAMARAO NARAYANA MURTHY

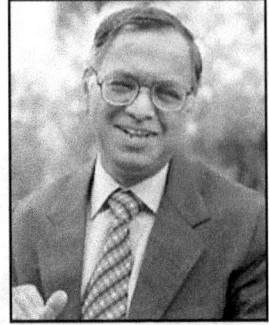

Nagavara Ramarao Narayana Murthy, better known as N. R. Narayana Murthy was born on August 20, 1946 in Mysore, Karnataka. He graduated with a degree in electrical engineering from the National Institute of Engineering, University of Mysore in 1967. He received his master's degree from IIT Kanpur in 1969.

Mr. Murthy's first job position was at IIM Ahmedabad, where he worked as the chief systems programmer. He developed a time-sharing system and designed and implemented a BASIC interpreter for ECIL (Electronics Corporation of India Limited). After IIM Ahmedabad, he started a company named *Softronics* in 1976. When that company failed, he joined the Patni Computer Systems in Pune. Mr. Murthy met his wife, Sudha Murthy in Pune who was an engineer working at Tata Engineering and Locomotive Co. Ltd. (Telco, now known as Tata Motors) at the time.

After settling down in Pune, Mr. Murthy founded *Infosys* in 1981 with an initial capital injection of Rs. 10,000, which was invested by his wife Sudha Murty. Murthy served as the CEO of Infosys for 21 years and was succeeded by co-founder Nandan Nilekani in 2002. At Infosys, he articulated, designed and implemented the Global Delivery Model which has become the foundation for the huge success in IT services outsourcing from India. He also lead the company through several key decisions including its listing on the Indian Stock Exchange and on the NASDAQ.

He held the executive position of the Chairman of the Board from 2002 to 2006, when he became the "non-executive" Chairman of the Board and Chief Mentor. In August 2011, he retired completely from the company and took the title, 'Chairman Emeritus'.

Trivia

Murthy is the brother-in-law of serial entrepreneur Gururaj "Desh" Deshpandey.

Quote

"The real power of money is the power to give it away."

🎥 🎥

STEVE JOBS

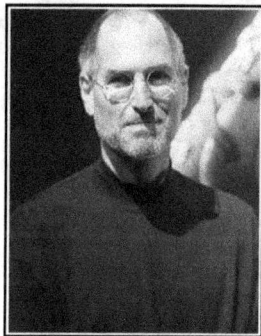

Born on February 24, 1955, Steven Paul 'Steve' Jobs was an American inventor and businessman. He was the Co-founder, Chairman, and Chief Executive Officer of Apple Inc.

In the late 1970s, Jobs, along with Apple co-founder Steve Wozniak, Mike Markkula and others designed, developed and marketed one of the first commercially successful lines of personal computers, the Apple II series.

In the early 1980s, Jobs was among the first to see the commercial potential of Xerox PARC's mouse-driven graphical user interface, which led to the creation of the Apple Lisa and, one year later, the Macintosh. After losing a power struggle with the board of directors in 1985, Jobs left Apple and founded a computer platform development company specialising in business markets, 'NeXT'.

Apple's 1996 buyout of 'NeXT' brought Jobs back to the company he co-founded and he served as its interim CEO from 1997, then becoming the permanent CEO in 2000, spearheading the advent of the iPod, iPhone and iPad.

From 2003, he was fighting an eight-year battle with cancer and eventually, resigned as CEO in August 2011, while on his third medical leave. He was then elected as Chairman of Apple's board of directors.

On October 5, 2011, around 3:00 p.m., Jobs died at his home in Palo Alto, California, aged 56, six weeks after resigning as CEO of Apple.

Trivia

Jobs was born in San Francisco and adopted at birth by Paul Jobs and Clara Jobs. When asked about his 'adoptive parents', Jobs replied emphatically that Paul and Clara Jobs 'were my parents'. He later stated in his authorised biography that they 'were my parents 1,000 percent".

🎥 🎥

HISTORIANS & HISTORIC FIGURES

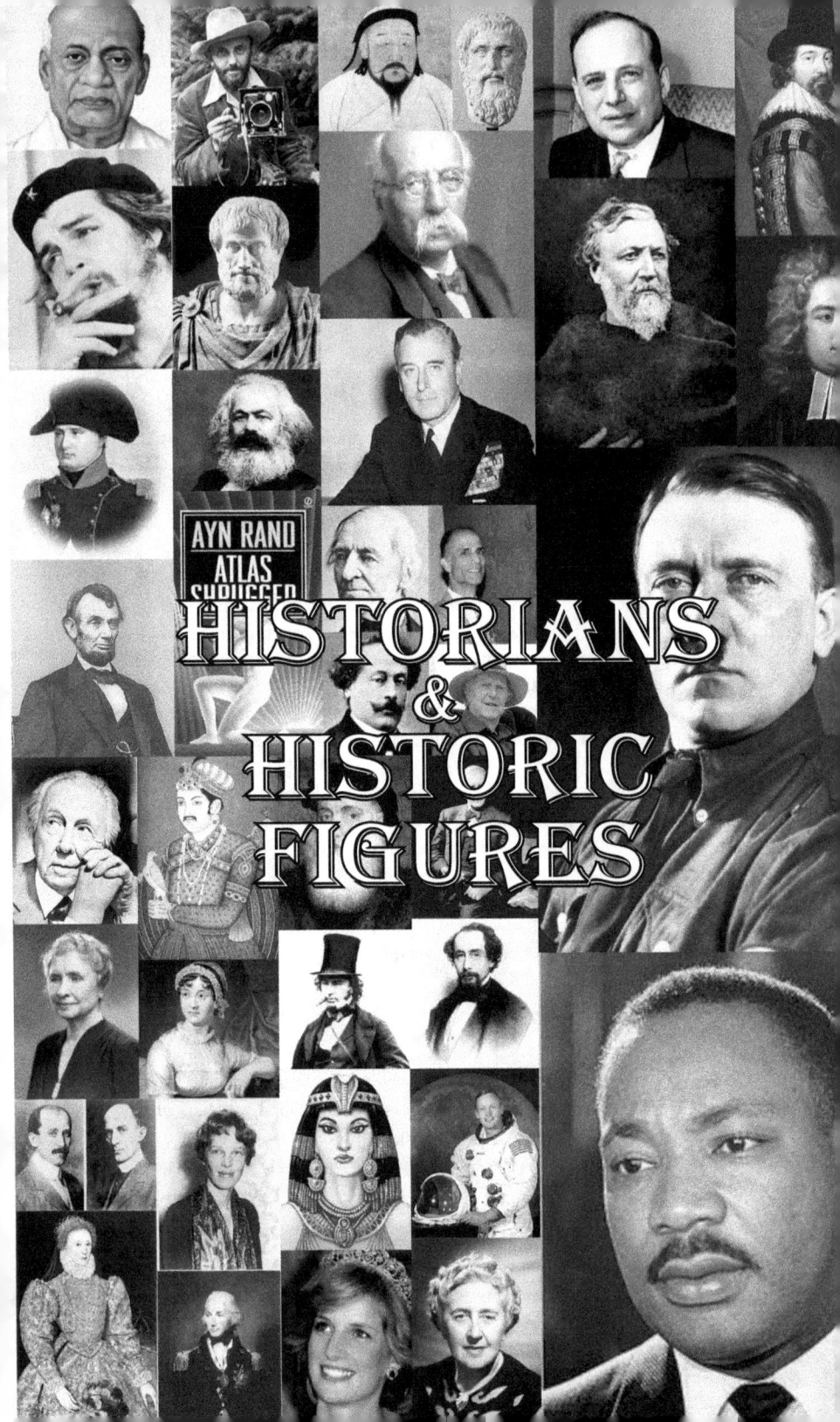

AYN RAND
ATLAS SHRUGGED

ABRAHAM LINCOLN

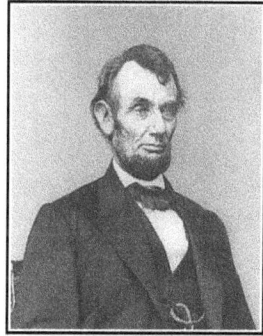

An American hero, Abraham Lincoln is still remembered across the world as the one who rose from being ordinary to extraordinary. He was the President of the United States from 1861 to 1865 and a saviour of those enslaved.

Born in Hodgeville, Kentucky, Lincoln grew up on his father's farm. He used to help his father to look after the crops in the farm. He did meagre chores like splitting fence rails and working in a general store as a clerk. Whatever knowledge he acquired was from the books he read in the time he got between his chores.

This self-gathered education enabled him to become one of the finest lawyers of the world and the **President of The United States**.

In 1842, he married Mary Anne Todd and had four sons. However, only one of them survived.

An actor, John Wilkes Booth, shot Lincoln on April 14, 1865, while he was on a visit to the Ford's Theatre. He passed away after being in coma for long and became the first   S President to be ever assassinated.

As the President of he guided the people during the Civil War. He issued the **Emancipation Proclamation** in 1863 to free people from slavery. His famous **Gettysburg Address** is still remembered and is quoted as the best speech in the history of America. He shed his views on the need for a free world with no bias towards any race.

Trivia

On Abraham Lincoln's 100th birthday in 1909, a penny was issued with his face on it to commemorate the occasion, becoming the first American coin to bear a president's image on it.

Quote

"As I would not be a slave, so I would not be a master. This expresses my idea of democracy."

33

AKBAR

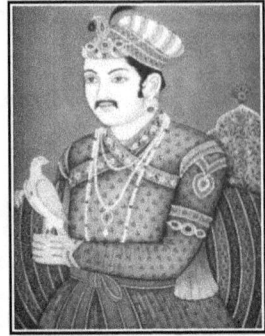

The third Mughal Emperor of India, Jalaluddin Muhammad Akbar is known for the rich cultural tradition India enjoys today.

Being forced into exile by the Afghan leader, Sher Shah Suri, Akbar's father, Emperor Humayun was on the run in 1540 when Akbar was born to him and his wife, Begum Hamida Banu on October 15, 1542, in Sind.

Therefore, Akbar spent most of his childhood running and fighting and hence, couldn't get any formal education. But, this did not hamper his interest in art, architecture, literature and music.

Humayun recaptured Delhi in 1555. Akbar was entitled to the throne after his sudden death. Akbar took full control as the King in 1560 and died on October 17, 1605.

As an emperor, Akbar conquered the whole of Hindustan (India). He amalgamated the Hindus and Muslims by removing the *jizya* (tax) that the non-Muslims had to pay.

He married a Rajput princesses, making it possible for the Hindus to be a part of the ruling dynasty.

He banned cow slaughter and allowed the Jesuits to build a church in Agra. He built a place of worship in Fatehpur Sikri where people of all religions were invited.

He held an open court session every week to know about the problems faced by them. His court consisted of a group of 'nine extraordinary people' called the *Navratnas*, meaning 'nine jewels'.

Ain-i-Akbari and *Akbarnama*, the two very important historical works, were written by Abul Fazal in Akbar's honour.

Trivia

Akbar created a new religion called Din-i-Ilahi in 1581, as he believed that one religion did not had the sole authority over truth. The new religion promoted ethics, discouraged sins and held virtues, such as kindness and prudence as its core.

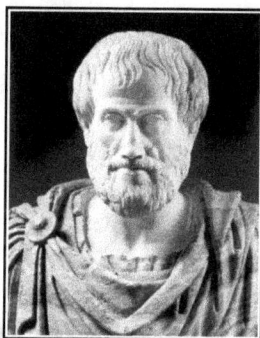

ARISTOTLE

Aristotle, one of Plato's greatest disciples, was born in 384 BC. He was a Greek philosopher and a polymath.

Aristotle's father was a physician to the king of Macedonia. His father sent Aristotle to study at the academy when he was seven years old.

At the beginning, he was there as a student, then became a researcher and finally a teacher. He adopted and developed Platonic ideas there. When Plato died, Plato willed the Academy to his nephew, Speusippus and not to Aristotle.

Aristotle then went to Assos in Asia Minor to open a branch of the Academy. This particular Academy focused more on biology than its predecessor that relied on mathematics.

His writings covered many subjects – rhetoric, metaphysics, physics, poetry, music, theatre, politics, logic, linguistics, government, biology, ethics, and zoology.

He married the niece of another former student of Plato, Hermias. Pythias died after Pythias, ten years. During these years in Assos, Aristotle started to break away from Platonism and developed his own ideas.

Later, Aristotle was invited by King Philip of Macedonia in 343 BC to tutor his thirteen-ear-old don, Alexander.

King Philip was then murdered in 336 BC after which Alexander became the king. He mobilised his father's great army and subdued some city-states, thus becoming 'Alexander The Great'.

After Aristotle stopped teaching Alexander the Great, he returned to Athens in 335 BC.

Then, Aristotle founded his own school, which was named the Lyceum, named after the Greek God, Apollo Lyceus.

He died in Athens in 322 BC.

Trivia

Aristotle's works that have survived from antiquity through medieval manuscript transmission are collected in the Corpus Aristotelicum.

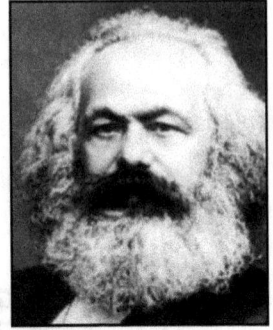

KARL MARX

A Philosopher, social scientist, historian and revolutionary, Karl Marx, is without a doubt the most influential socialist thinker to emerge in the 19th century. Born on May 5, 1818, Karl Marx developed the socio-political theory of Marxism.

Karl Heinrich Marx was born into a comfortable middle-class family in Trier on the river Moselle in Germany. At the age of 17, Marx enrolled in the Faculty of Law at the University of Bonn. Then, he went to the University of Berlin.

In 1836, he got engaged to Jenny von Westphalen and married her in 1843. Marx moved into journalism after his studies and in October 1842, became editor of the influential *Rheinische Zeitung*, which was a liberal newspaper backed by industrialists. The Prusssian government closed the paper due to his articles.

Moving to Paris in 1843, Karl Marx began writing for other radical newspapers including the *Deutsch-Französische Jahrbücher* and *Vorwärts*. He also wrote a series of books, several of which were co-written with his fellow German revolutionary socialist, Friedrich Engels. His most notable books were *The Communist Manifesto* and *Capital.*

After Marx was expelled from Paris at the end of 1844, he moved to Brussels. Marx became a communist and set down his views in his writings known as the **Economic and Philosophical Manuscripts** in 1844, which remained unpublished until the 1930s.

His other major contributions were *The German Ideology, The Communist Manifesto, The Class Struggles in France* and *The 18th Brumaire of Louis Bonaparte.*

Marx died on March 14, 1883 after prolonged illness.

Trivia

He was not a very well-known figure during his life, but his works became popular soon after his death.

MARTIN LUTHER KING

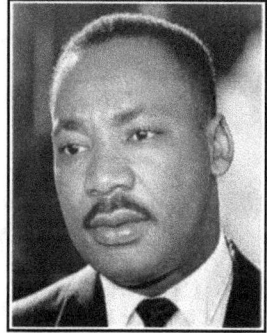

Martin Luther King Jr. was born on January 15, 1929 in Atlanta, Georgia. His father, Martin Luther King Sr., was a pastor of the Ebenezer Baptist Church in Atlanta. His mother was a schoolteacher.

After graduating from Morehouse College at the age of 19, he decided to enter Crozer Theological Seminary in Chester, Pennsylvania. He won the highest class ranking and a $1,200 fellowship for graduate school. In 1951, he entered the Boston University School of Theology to pursue his Ph.D.

He led the 1955 Montgomery Bus Boycott and helped found the Southern Christian Leadership Conference in 1957, serving as its first president. King's efforts led to the 1963 March on Washington, where King delivered his "I Have a Dream" speech. There, he expanded American values to include the vision of a colour blind society, and established his reputation as one of the greatest orators in American history.

Martin became the youngest person to receive the **Nobel Peace Prize** in 1964 for his work to end racial segregation and racial discrimination through civil disobedience and other non-violent means. By the time of his death in 1968, he had refocused his efforts on ending poverty and stopping the Vietnam War.

King was assassinated on April 4, 1968, in Memphis, Tennessee. He was posthumously awarded the 'Presidential Medal of Freedom' in 1977 and 'Congressional Gold Medal' in 2004. Martin Luther King. Jr. Day was established as a U.S. federal holiday in 1986.

Trivia

January 20, 1986 was the first national celebration of King's birthday as a holiday.

Quote

"Be a sinner and sin strongly, but more strongly have faith and rejoice in Christ."

NAPOLEON

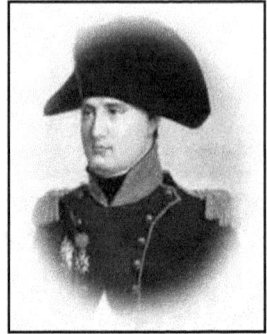

Napoleon was born on August 15, 1769 in Corsica to parents of noble Genoese ancestry and trained as an artillery officer in mainland France. He rose to prominence under the French First Republic and led successful campaigns against the First and Second Coalitions arrayed against France. In 1799, he staged a coup d'état and installed himself as the First Consul; five years later the French Senate proclaimed him Emperor.

In the first decade of the 19th century, the French Empire under Napoleon engaged in a series of conflicts – *the Napoleonic Wars* – involving every major European power. After a streak of victories, France secured a dominant position in continental Europe, and Napoleon maintained the French sphere of influence through the formation of extensive alliances and the appointment of friends and family members to rule other European countries as French client states. Napoleon's campaigns are studied at military academies throughout the world.

The fight against the guerrilla in Spain and 1812 French invasion of Russia marked turning points in Napoleon's fortunes. His Grande Armée was badly damaged in the campaign and never fully recovered. Napoleon spent the last six years of his life in confinement by the British on the island of Saint Helena. An autopsy concluded that he died of stomach cancer, although this claim has sparked significant debate, and some scholars have held that he was a victim of arsenic poisoning.

Trivia
He is famed for his great military successes.

Quote
"A leader is a dealer in hope."

PLATO

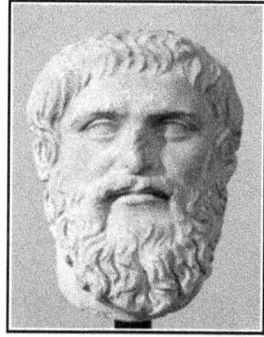

Born around 428 BCE in Athens, Plato was a Classical Greek philosopher, student of Socrates, mathematician, writer of philosophical dialogues and founder of the Academy in Athens.

Plato's father died while he was very young and his mother remarried to Pyrilampes.

He studied music and poetry at a very young age. Plato developed the foundations of his metaphysics and epistemology by studying the doctrines of Cratylus, and the work of Pythagoras and Parmenides, according to Aristotle.

Later, Plato adopted his philosophy and style of debate as Socrates' disciple. Plato was in military service from 409 BC to 404 BC. Socrates' execution in 399 BC had a profound effect on Plato.

Plato began to write extensively after 399 BC. Most scholars agree to divide Plato's major work into three distinct groups. The first of these is known as the *Socratic Dialogues* because of how close he stays within the text to Socrates' teachings.

Other texts relegated to this group include the Crito, Laches, Lysis, Charmides, Euthyphro, and Hippias Minor and Major.

The period from 387 to 361 BC is often called Plato's 'middle' or transitional period. It is thought that he may have written the Meno, Menexenus, Cratylus, Euthydemus, Phaedrus, Repuglic, Syposium and Phaedo during this time.

Plato's most influential work, *The Republic,* is also a part of his middle dialogues.

Plato died in 347 BC, leaving his school of learning Academy to his sister's son, Speusippus. The Academy remained a model for institutions of higher learning until it was closed in 529 CE.

Trivia

Plato's birth name was Aristocles, and he gained the nickname, Platon, meaning broad, because of his broad build.

QUEEN ELIZABETH

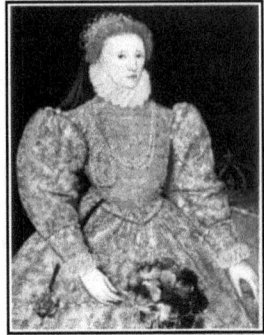

Born on September 7, 1533, Elizabeth I is considered to be one of the greatest monarchs of England and Ireland from November 17, 1558 until her death.

Sometimes called Gloriana, The Virgin Queen, Elizabeth was the fifth and last monarch of the Tudor dynasty. Daughter of Henry VIII, she was born a princess. Her mother, Anne Boleyn was executed two and a half years after her birth and Elizabeth was declared illegitimate.

In 1558, Elizabeth succeeded the Catholic Mary I, during whose reign she had been imprisoned for nearly a year on suspicion of supporting protestant rebels.

Elizabeth was more moderate than her father, brother and sister had been, in her government. One of her mottoes was 'video et taceo' (I see, and say nothing). After 1570, when the pope declared her illegitimate, several conspiracies threatened her life. However, all plots were defeated with the help of her ministers' secret service.

Elizabeth was cautious in foreign affairs, moving between the major powers of France and Spain. The defeat of the Spanish Armada in the mid 1580s, when they tried to conquer England, associated her with what is popularly viewed as one of the greatest victories in English history.

She died on March 24, 1603.

Trivia

It was expected that Elizabeth would marry and produce an heir so as to continue the Tudor line. But not doing so, as she grew older, Elizabeth became famous for her virginity and a cult grew up around her which was celebrated in the portraits, pageants and literature of the day.

SUBHAS CHANDRA BOSE

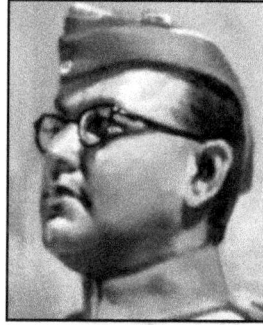

Subhas Chandra Bose was born on January 23, 1897 in Cuttack, Orissa to Janakinath Bose and Prabhabati Devi.

Known by the name, Netaji, Subhas Chandra Bose was an Indian revolutionary, who led an Indian national political and military force against Britain and the Western powers during the World War II.

Being one of the most prominent leaders in the Indian independence movement, he is a legendary figure in India

He is presumed to have died on August 18, 1945, from injuries sustained in an alleged aircraft crash in Taihoku Taipei. However, no actual evidence of his death on that day has been authenticated. Many committees were set up by the government of India to investigate the mystery of his presumed death.

Subhas Chandra Bose advocated complete unconditional independence for India, whereas, the All-India Congress Committee wanted it in phases. Later, at the historic Lahore Congress convention, the Congress adopted *Purna Swaraj* (complete independence) as its motto. Subhas Chandra Bose later wrote that the great enthusiasm he saw among the people enthused him tremendously and that he doubted if any other leader anywhere in the world received such a reception as Gandhi did during these travels across the country.

Trivia

He was imprisoned and expelled from India. He came back to India and was imprisoned again for defying the ban.

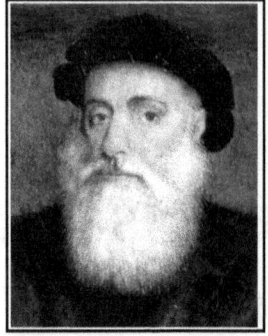

VASCO DA GAMA

Born in 1460, Vasco da Gama was a Portuguese navigator and acquired a reputation as a brave and able sea commander. When the king of Portugal decided to send an expedition in search of a passage south of Africa to India, Vasco da Gama was selected to command.

After confessing and receiving absolution after the manner of those going to their death, Vasco and his companions set out with four ships. In spite of storms and tempests, they reached Calicut, and set up a marble pillar in evidence of their arrival in the country.

A fleet of 13 ships was sent out at once to establish a factory for trade with India. The ships returned in due time, heavily laden with rich shawls, silks, spices and precious gems bringing great gain into the king's coffers.

In 1502, he was sent accordingly with a fleet to the coast of India. He bombarded Calicut and treated the inhabitants with great cruelty.

He was made the Portuguese Viceroy of India.

He died in India on December 24, 1524 and was buried in a monastery, but his remains were brought home and buried with pomp and ceremony.

Trivia

He was instrumental in making Portugal for a time the leading commercial nation of Europe.

Quote

"May God our Lord allow us to complete our journey in His service, Amen."

SINGERS/
MUSICIANS

A.R. RAHMAN

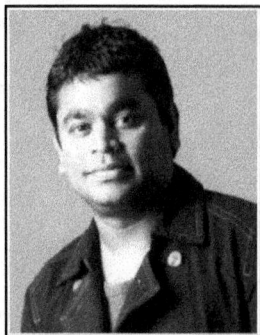

Allah Rakha Rahman (A.R. Rahman) was born on January 6, 1966 in Madras, presently Chennai as A.S. Dileep Kumar. He is an Indian music composer, record producer, musician, singer and philanthropist. Rahman started learning piano at the age of four. His father passed away when he was nine years old.

He accompanied the great tabla maestro, Zakir Hussain on a few world tours and also won a scholarship at the 'Trinity College of Music' at Oxford University.

Then he moved to advertising and composed more than 300 jingles over five years. In 1989, he started a small studio called the Panchathan Record Inn that was one of the most well-equipped and advanced sound recording studios in India.

Rahman played a few of his music samples to famous director Mani Ratnam at an award function and Mani Ratnam took him as a music composer in his next film – *Roja*. The enormous success of his first Hindi venture was followed by the chart-topping soundtrack albums.

A.R. Rahman now is popularly known as the man who has redefined contemporary Indian music. Hailed by the *Time* magazine as the 'Mozart of Madras', Rahman, according to a BBC estimate, has sold more than 150 million copies of his work comprising music from more than 100 film soundtracks and albums across over half a dozen languages, including landmark scores, such as 'Roja', 'Bombay', Dil Se', 'Taal', 'Lagaan', 'Vandemataram' and more recently, 'Jodhaa Akbar', 'Delhi 6' and 'Slumdog Millionaire'.

In 2009, Rahman bagged two Occars for his work in *Slumdog Millionaire*.

Trivia

In 1989, Rahman converted to Islam, the religion of his mother's family.

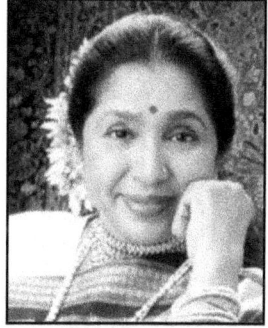

ASHA BHOSLE

A sha Bhosle was born on September 8, 1933 in a Marathi family. She is one of the best-known and most highly-regarded Hindi playback singers in India. She is sister of another legendary singer, Lata Mangeshkar.

Her career started in 1943 and spanned over six decades. She has sung songs for a number of Bollywod movies. Bhosle has sung over **12,000** songs, including pop music, ghazals, bhajans, traditional Indian classical music, folk songs and others.

She was conferred with the **Dadasaheb Phalke Award** in 2000 and the **Padma Vibhushan** in 2008. 'The World Records Academy' recognised her as the 'Most Recorded Artist' in 2009. In 2011, she was officially acknowledged by the Guinness Book of World Records as the most recorded artist.

She has been a versatile singer throughout her career. Be it the romantic, 'Oh Mere Sona Re' or the sensuous, 'Aaiye Meherban' or the peppy, 'Kambakth Ishq', Asha Bhosle has been adding life to every song.

Being a renowned singer and actor, her father, Dinanath Mangeshkar, trained her in classical music at a very young age.

Asha got a chance to sing in a Marathi film at the age of ten. After a lot of struggle, Asha did playback singing for Hindi movie, *Chunariya* in 1948.

She eloped with her sister, Lata Mangeshkar's Personal Secretary Ganpatrao Bhosle at the age of 16 and married him. The marriage didn't work and she came back to her maternal house with her children. In 1980, she married music director RD Burman.

The movie, *Teesri Manzil* released in 1966 gave her enormous fame and she was acclaimed all over India and abroad as well.

Trivia

Asha Bhosle is a successful restaurateur and runs a chain of restaurants in Dubai and Kuwait, called the Asha's.

BISMILLAH KHAN

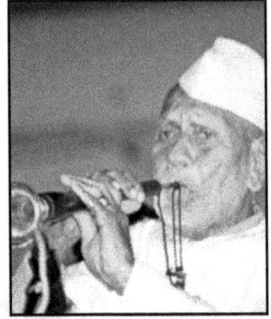

Ustad Bismillah Khan was born on March 21, 1916 in Dumraon, Bihar. He was the second son of Paigambar Khan and Mitthan. The *shehnai* maestro was a **Bharat Ratna** Awardee and has been also awarded other three top Civilian Awards – **Padma Shri**, **Padma Bhushan** and **Padma Vibhushan**.

He gained worldwide acclaim for playing the shehnai for more than eight decades. He was named Qamaruddin to sound like his elder brother's name Shamsuddin. But, when his grandfather Rasool Baksh Khan saw him as a baby, he uttered the word 'Bismillah' and hence he came to be known as Bismillah Khan.

He moved to Varanasi at the age of six. He received his training under his uncle, late Ali Baksh 'Vilayatu', who was also a shehnai player. He mastered the art soon and is credited for making shehnai as one of the Indian classical instruments.

His concert in All India Music Conference in 1937 in Calcutta (Kolkata) brought shehnai into limelight and was hugely appreciated by music lovers.

Bismillah Khan had the rare honour of playing his shehnai on the eve of India's independence in 1947 and has been performing at the Red Fort since that year on August 15. He has a huge fan following across the world.

Ustaad Sahab Bismillah Khan died on August 21, 2006 at the age of 90 due to a cardiac arrest. His shehnai was buried with him in his grave.

Trivia

He started calling his Shehnai as 'Begum' after his wife died.

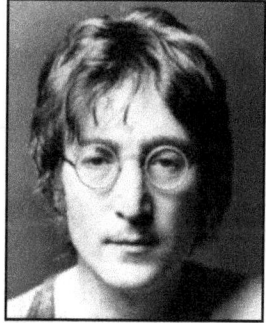

JOHN LENNON

John Winston Lennon (October 9, 1940 – December 8, 1980) was an English musician and singer-songwriter.

Lenon rose to worldwide fame being among the founding members of one of the most commercially successful and critically acclaimed acts in the history of popular music, *The Beatles*.

He and **Paul McCartney** formed one of the most successful song-writing partnerships of the 20th century.

Born and raised in Liverpool, Lennon's first band The Quarrymen evolved into The Beatles in 1960.

After the group disintegrated towards the end of the decade, Lennon embarked on a solo career that produced the critically acclaimed albums 'John Lennon/Plastic Ono Band' and 'Imagine' and iconic songs, such as 'Give Peace a Chance' and 'Imagine'. He married Yoko Ono in 1969 and changed his name to John Ono Lennon.

In 1975, Lennon disengaged himself from the music business to devote time to his son, Sean but re-emerged in 1980s with a new album, 'Double Fantasy'.

Lenon was murdered three weeks after the album was released.

Lennon gave a sense of a rebellious nature in his music, his drawing, his writing, on film, and in interviews, which made him controversial. He moved to New York City in 1971, where his criticism of the Vietnam War resulted in a lengthy attempt by Richard Nixon's administration to deport him, but his songs were adopted as *anthems* by the anti-war movement.

Trivia

As of 2010 data, Lennon's solo album sales in the US exceed 14 million units. As a writer, co-writer or performer, he is responsible for 25 number-one singles on the US Hot 100 chart.

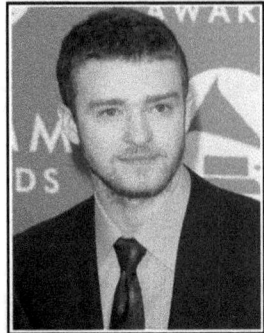

JUSTIN TIMBERLAKE

Justin Randall Timberlake was born to Lynn Harless and Randy Timberlake on January 31, 1981 in Memphis, Tennessee.

Timberlake grew up singing in the church choir. From 1993 to 1995, he performed with The Mickey Mouse Club along with pop stars, Britney Spears, Christina Aguilera and JC Chasez.

At the age of 14, Justin became a member of the boy band, *NSYNC. The group released their self-titled debut album in 1998. They became popular with fans and made a place for themselves in the music industry with a succession of big-selling albums.

Justin usually spent time working on and writing songs for his debut solo album in the beginning of 2002. During this time, he broke up with his longtime girlfriend, Britney Spears. His first solo album titled 'Justified' was released in 2002. His songs from his solo album debuting at number one of the music charts include 'SexyBack', 'My Love', and 'What Goes Around, Comes Around' from his second successful album, 'Future Sex/Love Sounds' in 2006.

He also has an acting career having starred in films, such as *The Social Network*, *Bad Teacher* and *Friends with Benefits*.

His other ventures include record label, Tennman Records, fashion label William Rast and the restaurants, Destino and Southern Hospitality.

Timberlake has won **six Grammy Awards** and **four Emmy Awards**.

Trivia
When he is not able to fall asleep, he sings himself to sleep.

Quote
"I'm a perfectionist. I can't help it, I get really upset with myself if I fail in the least."

🎥 🎥

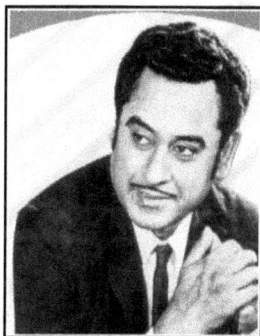

KISHORE KUMAR

Born as Abhas Kumar Ganguly on August 4, 1929, the great singer, popularly known as Kishore Kumar and affectionately called Kishore Da, was one of those very few singers who took risks and experimented with different styles of music.

Kishore was the youngest in the Ganguly family and preferred singing and mimicking, Kundanlal Saigal. Once SD Burman had come to Ashok Kumar's house to meet him when he heard Kishore Kumar singing. He actually thought it was Saigal singing and inquired if he was there too. When he came to know that it was Kishore singing, he appreciated and encouraged young Kishore to continue refining his voice but at the same time, develop a style of his own. He, then, developed his own *signature style*.

He perfected *yodelling*. In Hindi film industry, his yodelling turned out to be widely popular and became a trademark of Kishore Kumar. His songs sounded absolutely natural, like laughter.

Kishore Kumar used to incorporate non-sensical terms into his songs that gave it an entirely a new feel. The ability to transform his voice according to not just the scene, but also the actor is something that was truly incredible of Kishore. He has sung many songs for Bollywood films. He has sung soulful songs for Dev Anand and also fun-filled songs for Rajesh Khanna, the yesteryear superstar.

Kishore Da has given some timeless classics, such as 'Chalte Chalte Mere Yeh Geet', 'Ek Ladki Bhigi Bhagi Si', 'Koi Humdum Na Raha', 'Yeh Jeevan Hai' and many others till his last song, 'Guru Guru Aajao Sanam'.

He was at the peak of his filmi career in 70's and 80's and died on October 13, 1987.

Trivia

Kishore Kumar had put a sign of 'Beware of Kishore' outside one of his flats, where he stayed for some time while his bungalow was made up.

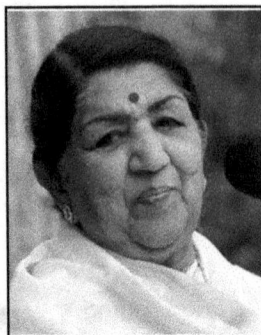

LATA MANGESHKAR

Popularly known as the 'Nightingale of India', Lata Mangeshkar is the most versatile and popular playback singer of Hindi cinema, and was a theatre artist as well.

Born on September 28, 1929 in Indore, she started working as a theatre artist in *sangeet nataks* at the age of five. Being the first child of Dinanath Mangeshkar, she is the elder sister of singer Asha Bhosle.

She started learning music from her father Dinanath. Lata Mangeshkar began her career in 1942 which spanned over six and a half decades.

She sang songs in Hindi and about thirty-six other regional Indian languages and foreign languages.

After the sudden death of her father Dinanath, she decided to play small roles in various Hindi and Marathi films due to unsound financial condition of the house.

Lata got her biggest break when she was given a chance to sing the song 'Aayega Aanewaala' for the movie, *Mahal.* Her career saw a tremendous growth in the 1950s. She has worked with all the renowned music composers of her time like Shankar Jaikishan, SD Burman, Salil Chowdhury, Naushad, Hemant Kumar, etc.

She has sung songs for popular films like *Lamhe, Diwale Dulhaniya Le Jayenge, Darr, Yeh Dillagi, Dil toh Pagal Hai,* etc.

She has won several awards including the **Padma Bhushan, Dada Saheb Phalke Award, Padma Vibhushna** for her singing. She is also been conferred with India's highest civilian award, the **Bharat Ratna.**

Trivia

Lata Mangeshkar has composed music and also produced movies under the name of 'Anand Ghan'. She is very fond of cooking. She always sings barefoot, in studies or on the stage.

LUCIANO

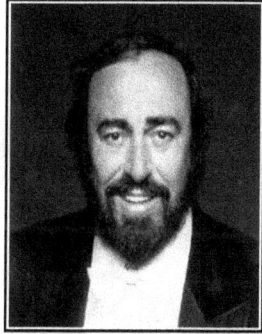

Luciano was born on October 12, 1935, in Modena, Emilia-Romagna, in Northern Italy. His father, Fernando Pavarotti, was a gifted amateur tenor, who instilled a love for music and singing in young Luciano. His mother, Adele Venturi, worked at the local cigar factory. Young Pavarotti showed many talents. He first sang with his father in the Corale Rossi, a male choir in Modena, and won the first prize in an international choir competition in Wales, UK. He also played soccer as a goalkeeper for his town's junior team.

Pavarotti made his operatic debut on April 29, 1961, as Rodolfo in La Boheme by Giacomo Puccini, at the opera house in Reggio, Emilia. Eventually, Pavarotti stepped in for Di Stefano in 1963, at the Royal Opera House in London as 'Rodolfo' in La Boheme by Giacomo Puccini, making his international debut. Pavarotti made his American debut opposite Sutherland in February of 1965, in Miami Opera. In March 2004, Pavarotti gave his last performance in an opera as painter Mario Cavaradossi in Giacomo Puccini's 'Tosca' at the New York Metropolitan Opera.

Luciano Pavarotti died of kidney failure on September 6, 2007, at home in Modena, Italy, where he was surrounded by his family. He was laid to eternal rest with his parents in the family tomb in Montale Rangone cemetery near Modena. His funeral ceremony in Modena was an international event attended by celebrities and over fifty thousand music lovers from all over the world.

Trivia
He was a recipient of the 'John F. Kennedy Center Honors' in 2001.

Quote
"Above all, I am an opera singer. This is how people will remember me."

MADONNA

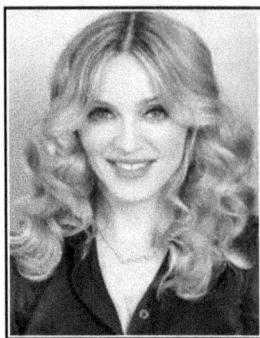

Madonna was born on August 16, 1958. She is an American singer-songwriter, actress and entrepreneur. Throughout her career, many of her songs have hit number one on the record charts, including "Like a Virgin", "Papa Don't Preach", "Like a Prayer", "Vogue", "Frozen", "Music", "Hung Up", and "4 Minutes". Critics have praised Madonna for her diverse musical productions, while at the same time serving as a lightning rod for religious controversy.

She won critical acclaim and a **Golden Globe** Award for Best Actress in Motion Picture Musical or Comedy for her role in *Evita* (1996), but has received harsh feedback for her other film roles. Madonna's other ventures include being a fashion designer, children's book author, film director and producer. Madonna has been acclaimed as a businesswoman. In 1992, she founded the entertainment company *Maverick* as a joint venture with the 'Time Warner'. In 2007, she signed an unprecedented US $120 million contract with Live Nation.

Madonna has sold more than 300 million records worldwide and is recognised as the world's top-selling female recording artist of all time by the 'Guinness World Records', according to the Recording Industry Association of America (RIAA),

In 2008, *Billboard* magazine ranked Madonna at number two, behind only The Beatles, on the Billboard Hot 100 All-Time Top Artists, making her the most successful solo artist in the history of the Billboard chart. She was also inducted into the Rock and Roll Hall of Fame in the same year.

Trivia

Madonna owns a chihuahua named Chiquita.

Quote

"Poor is the man whose pleasures depend on the permission of another."

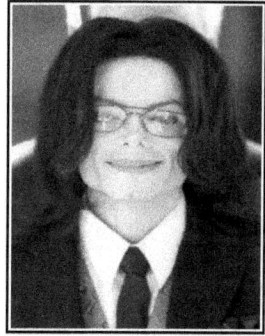

MICHAEL JACKSON

R eferred to as the 'King of Pop', American superstar Michael Jackson was born in Gary, Indiana, on August 29, 1958.

Popularly known as MJ, Jackson is recognised as the most successful entertainer of all time by the 'Guinness World Records'.

Michael Jackson started his career as a singer along with his brothers as a member of 'The Jackson 5'. Soon he became a well-known figure in the music industry due to his mature dance moves and voice.

The five brothers, Jackie, Tito, Jermaine, Michael and Marlon gave many chart-busting hits including 'I Want You Back', 'Never Can Say Goodbye', 'Got to Be There' and many others.

He started his inevitable solo career in 1971. He uneasily ventured into films like 'The Wiz' in 1978 but was more successful with his music videos.

Michael had two brief marriages. In May 1994, Jackson married Elvis Presley's daughter, Lisa Marie Presley and they got divorced in less than two years of their marriage.

Jackson, then, got married to his long-time friend, Deborah Jeanne Rowe. They had two children – Michael Joseph Jackson Jr (commonly known as Prince) and Paris-Michael Katherine Jackson. The couple divorced in 1999 and Jackson got full custody of the children.

Jackson's life has been full of controversies. He was accused of child sexual abuse in 1993 but the case was settled out of court. In 2005, he was tried and acquitted of other sexual abuse allegations after the jury ruled him not guilty.

For all it to end, he died of drug-induced cardiac arrest on June 25, 2009 when he was preparing for his concert in London.

Trivia

His 1982 album, 'Thriller' is the biggest selling album of all time with confirmed sales of over 47 million, and over an estimated 100 million copies worldwide.

Mozart

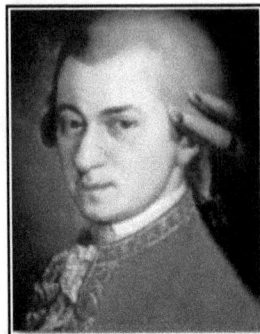

Mozart was born on January 27, 1756 in Salzburg, Austria. He grew up in Salzburg under the regulation of his strict father, Leopold who also was a famous composer of his time.

His abilities in music were obvious even when Mozart was still young so that in 1762 at the age of six, his father took him with his elder sister on a concert tour to Munich and Vienna and a second one from 1763-66 through the south of Germany, Paris and London. Mozart was celebrated as a wonder child everywhere because of his excellent piano playing and his improvisations.

In 1769, he became the concertmaster of the Archbishop and was knighted by the Pope in Rome. Working in Salzburg, he nevertheless travelled around Europe to meet other composers and orchestras. But in 1781, after a dispute with the Archbishop, he left Salzburg and went to Vienna, where he married Constanze Weber from Mannheim.

In Vienna, he also started his friendship with Joseph Haydn and a time of many work pieces. In the last year of his life, for example, he wrote one of his masterpieces, "Die Zauberflöte". Although some of his operas were successful, he could not make money from this and died in poverty at the age of 36, having even on his last day worked on a "Requiem". He was buried in a communal grave which could not be precisely identified years late .

Quote

"People are wrong who think my art comes easily to me. I assure you, nobody has devoted so much time and thought to composition as I."

USTAD AMJAD ALI KHAN

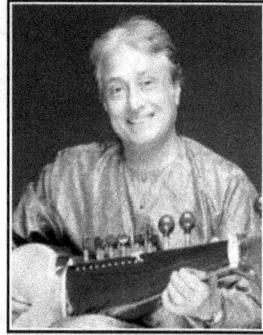

Born on October 9, 1945 in Gwalior, Ustad Amjad Ali Khan is a noted *sarod* player.

He belongs to the Bangash lineage and is the sixth generation sarod player in his family. He learnt sarod under his father, Haafiz Ali Khan's tutelage, who was also a musician to the royal family of Gwalior.

Amjad Ali Khan got the opportunity of his first solo recital at the age of 12 in 1958. Having developed a unique style of playing the sarod, he is considered one of the foremost classical musicians. The key innovations in his style are compositions based on vocal music, the technical ability to play highly complex phrases (ekhara taans) on the sarod spanning three octaves and the emphasis on simple and elegant compositions.

He has simplified the instrument by removing some strings and has also removed the resonant gourd (tumba) which is in use by the other sarod schools.

Amjad Ali Khan founded the Ustad Hafiz Ali Khan Memorial Society in 1977, which organises concerts and bestows an annual 'Hafiz Ali Khan Award'.

Ustad Amjad Ali Khan has performed in different parts of the world at various national and international festivals.

His family arranged a marriage for him, but that failed, and Khan got married second time to Bharatanatyam dancer Subhalakshmi in 1976. The couple has two sons – Amaan and Ayaan – who were taught music by their father.

He is the recipient of many awards and honours. These include: The **Padma Shri** (1975), **Sangeet Natak Academy Award** (1989), the **Tansen Award** (1989), the **Padma Bhushan** (1991) and the **International Music Forum Award**, UNESCO in 1970.

Trivia

Amjad Ali Khan is a Muslim and his wife, Subhalakshmi is a Hindu. Their family home in Gwalior was made into a musical centre and they live in New Delhi.

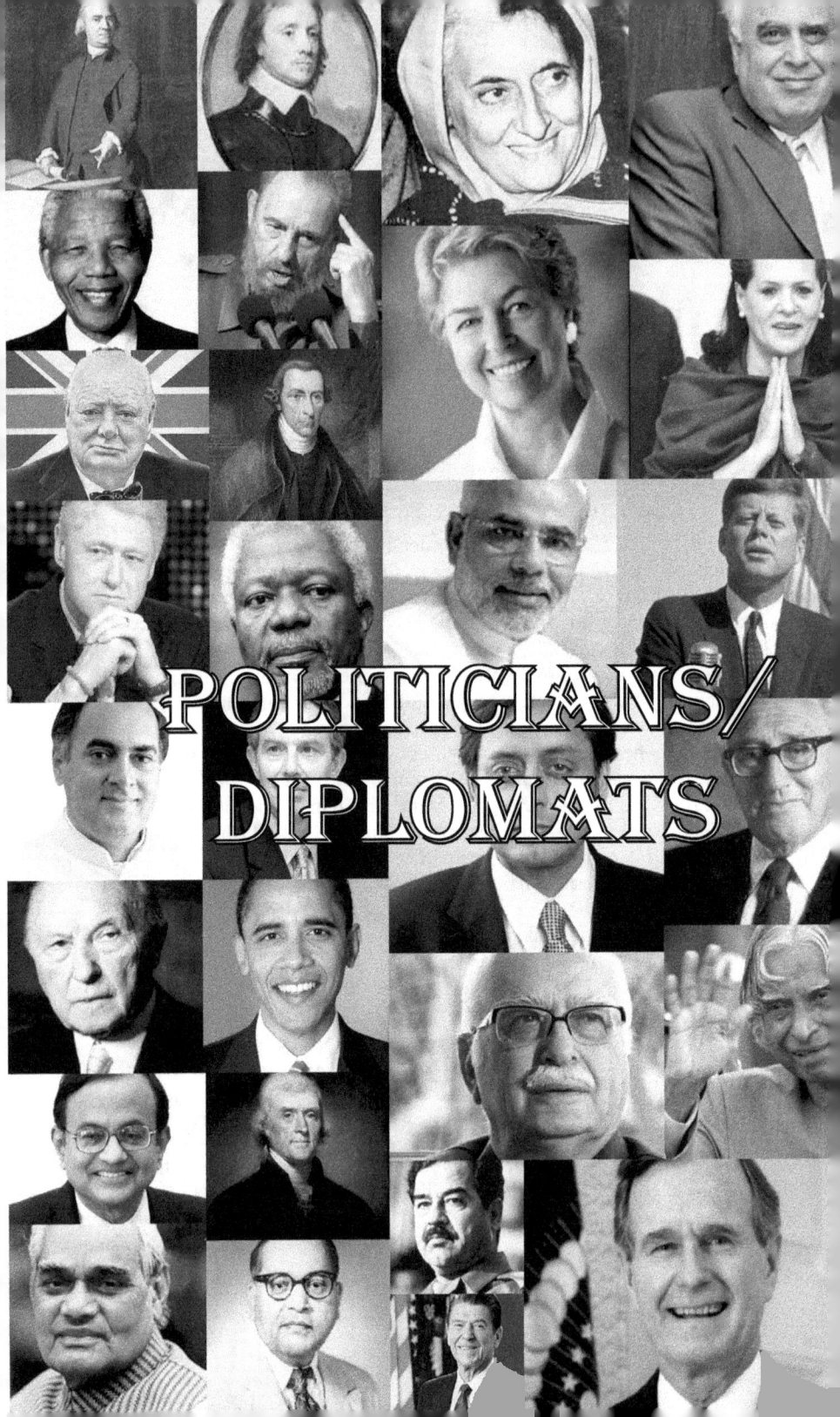

POLITICIANS/ DIPLOMATS

Anna Eleanor Roosevelt

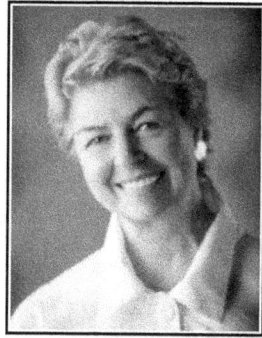

Anna Eleanor Roosevelt was born on October 11, 1884. She was the First Lady of the United States from 1933 to 1945. She supported the New Deal policies of her husband, distant cousin, Franklin Delano Roosevelt, and became an advocate for civil rights.

After her husband's death in 1945, Roosevelt continued to be an international author, speaker, politician, and activist for the 'New Deal Coalition'. She worked to enhance the status of working women, although she opposed the Equal Rights Amendment because she believed it would adversely affect women.

In the 1940s, Roosevelt was one of the co-founders of 'Freedom House' and supported the formation of the United Nations. Roosevelt founded the UN Association of the United States in 1943 to advance support for the formation of the UN. She was a delegate to the UN General Assembly from 1945 and 1952, a job for which she was appointed by President Harry S. Truman and confirmed by the United States Senate. During her time at the United Nations, she chaired the committee that drafted and approved the Universal Declaration of Human Rights. President Truman called her the "First Lady of the World" in tribute to her human rights achievements.

Active in politics for the rest of her life, Roosevelt chaired the John F. Kennedy administration's ground-breaking committee which helped start second-wave feminism, the Presidential Commission on the Status of Women. In 1999, she was ranked in the top ten of Gallup's List of Most Widely Admired People of the 20th Century.

Trivia
Roosevelt received 48 honorary degrees during her life.

Quote
"A little simplification would be the first step toward rational living, I think."

🎥 🎥

Atal Bihari Vajpayee

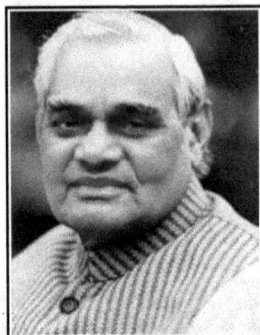

A tal Bihari Vajpayee was born to Krishna Devi and Krishna Bihari Vajpayee on December 25, 1924 in a Brahmin family in a town in Gwalior. Vajpayee's father Krishna Bihari was a poet and schoolmaster in his hometown.

Atal Bihari Vajpayee attended Gwalior's Victoria College, the present Laxmi Bai College, and graduated with distinctions in Hindi, English and Sanskrit. He did his Post Graduation in Political Science from the DAV College in Kanpur.

He started his career with joining the Rashtriya Swayamsevak Sangh (RSS), and served the *Rashtradharma, Veer Arjun* and *Panchjanya* newspapers as a journalist and poet.

Vajpayee never married, becoming the first and, till date, only bachelor Prime Minister of India.

After his first brief period as Prime Minister in 1996, Vajpayee headed a coalition government from March 19, 1998 till May 19, 2004.

Vajpaaye has been a parliamentarian for over four decades. He was elected to the Lok Sabha a record nine times and to the Rajya Sabha twice.

He was the Member of Parliament for Lucknow until 2009, when he retired from active politics due to health constraints.

Trivia

Vajpayee was referred to as 'The Bhishma Pitamah' of Indian Politics by Prime Minister Dr Manmohan Singh in one of his speeches.

Quote

"Global interdependence today means that economic disasters in developing countries could create a backlash on developed countries."

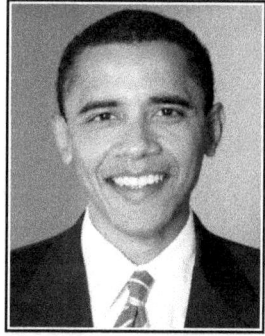

BARACK OBAMA

Barack Obama was born on August 4, 1961. Some of the nicknames given to him are 'Barry', 'Bama', 'Rock', 'The One', 'No drama Obama'. He was born to a white American mother, Ann Dunham and a black Kenyan father, Barack Obama Sr., who were both young college students at the University of Hawaii.

Obama attended the Columbia University but found New York's racial tension inescapable. He became a community organiser for a small Chicago church-based group for three years, helping poor South Side residents cope with a wave of plant closings. He then attended Harvard Law School, and in 1990 became the first African-American editor of the 'Harvard Law Review'.

He also began teaching at the University of Chicago Law School, and married Michelle Robinson, a fellow attorney. Eventually, he was elected to the Illinois state senate.

In 2004, Obama was elected to the US Senate as a Democrat, representing Illinois and he gained national attention by giving a rousing and well-received keynote speech at the Democratic National Convention in Boston. In 2008, he ran for President and despite having only four years of national political experience, he won. In January 2009, he was sworn in as the **44th President of the United States**, and *the first African-American* ever elected to that position. Obama was awarded the Nobel Peace Prize in 2009.

Trivia

He has won a Grammy for Best Spoken Word for the CD version of his autobiography, 'Dreams From My Father' (2006).

Quote

"Change will not come if we wait for some other person or some other time. We are the ones we've been waiting for. We are the change that we seek."

🎥 🎥

BILL CLINTON

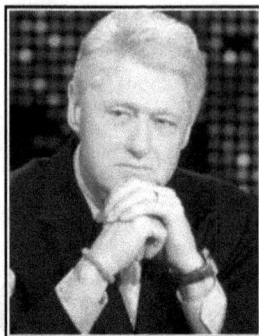

Born on August 19, 1946, William Jefferson 'Bill' Clinton is an American politician who served as the 42nd President of the United States from 1993 to 2001.

Bill Clinton was the third-youngest President. He took office as the President at the end of the Cold War. Bill Clinton was the first President of the baby boomer generation. Often described as a New Democrat, many of his policies have been attributed to a centrist, *Third Way philosophy of governance.*

Clinton became both a student leader and a skilled musician. An alumnus of Georgetown University, he earned a Rhodes scholarship to attend the University of Oxford. He is married to Hillary Rodham Clinton. Hillary Clinton was the Senator from New York from 2001 to 2009 and has been serving as the United States Secretary of State since 2009. Both Clintons received law degrees from Yale Law School, where they met and began dating.

Clinton was elected as the President in 1992, defeating incumbent President George HW Bush. As President, Clinton presided over the longest period of peacetime economic expansion in the history of America. He implemented Don't ask, don't tell, a controversial intermediate step to full gay military integration.

After a failed health care reform attempt, Republicans won control of Congress in 1994, for the first time in forty years. Two years later, the re-elected Clinton became the first member of the Democratic Party since Franklin D Roosevelt to win a second full term as President.

Trivia

As Governor of Arkansas, Bill Clinton overhauled the State's education system and served as Chair of the National Governors Association.

60

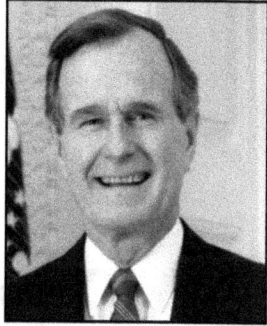

GEORGE H. W. BUSH

Born on June 12, 1924, George Herbert Walker Bush is an American politician who served as the 41st President of the United States (989–93). He had previously served as the 43rd Vice President of the United States from 1981 to 1989, a congressman, an ambassador and the Director of Central Intelligence.

Bush was born in Milton, Massachusetts, to Senator Prescott Bush and Dorothy Walker Bush. Following the attacks on Pearl Harbor in 1941, at the age of 18, Bush postponed going to college and became the youngest aviator in the US Navy at the time. He served until the end of the war, then attended the Yale University. Graduating in 1948, he moved his family to West Texas and entered the oil business, becoming a millionaire by the age of 40.

He became involved in politics soon after founding his own oil company, serving as a member of House of Representatives, among other positions. He ran unsuccessfully for president of the United States in 1980, but was chosen by party nominee Ronald Reagan to be the vice presidential nominee, and the two were subsequently elected. During his tenure, Bush headed administration task forces on deregulation and fighting drug abuse

Trivia

During the World War II, following the attack on Pearl Harbor in December 1941, Bush decided to join the US navy. So after graduating from the Phillips Academy, he became a naval aviator at the age of just 18!

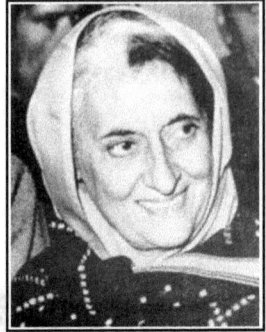

Indira Gandhi

Indira Priyadarshini Gandhi, known as Indira Gandhi, was born on November 19, 1917. She was an Indian politician who served as the Prime Minister of India for three consecutive terms – from 1966 to 1977 and a fourth term – 1980-1984.

Indira Gandhi was born to Jawaharlal and Kamala Nehru and spent her childhood in Allahabad. She received her college education at Somerville College, Oxford.

She married Feroze Gandhi in 1942 whom she knew from Allahabad and who died in 1960 before he could consolidate his own political force. The couple had two sons – **Rajiv Gandhi** and **Sanjay Gandhi**.

After the death of her father, Pt. Jawaharlal Nehru in 1964, Indira Gandhi was elected to Parliament and she was the Minister of Information and Broadcasting in Lal Bahadur Shastri's government. As Shastri died unexpectedly of a heart attack less than two years after assuming office, the numerous contenders for the position of the Prime Ministership picked Indira Gandhi as a compromise candidate. She showed extraordinary political skills and became the world's second longest serving female Prime Minister.

She was assassinated by her bodyguards as she garnered the undying hatred of Sikhs after she ordered an assault upon the Sikh shrine, the Golden Temple in Amritsar to crush the secessionist movement of Sikh militants, led by Jarnail Singh Bindranwale. The name of the operations was 'Operation Bluestar'.

Trivia

She was also the only Indian Prime Minister to have declared a state of emergency in order to 'rule by decree' and the only Indian Prime Minister to have been imprisoned after holding that office.

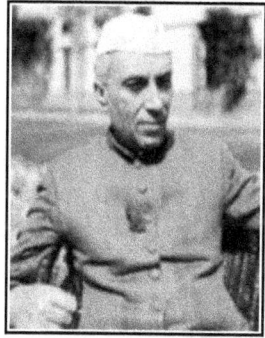

JAWAHARLAL NEHRU

Son of Swaroop Rani and Motilal Nehru, Jawaharlal Nehru was born on November 14, 1889, in Allahabad. Motilal Nehru was a wealthy lawyer and a prominent leader of the Indian independence movement.

Often referred as Panditji or affectionately *Chacha Nehru* by children, Nehru was the first Prime Minister of independent India from 1947 until he died on May 27, 1964.

He established the parliamentary government and became noted for his 'neutralist' policies in foreign affairs. He was also one of the principal leaders of India's independence movement in the 1930s and 1940s.

The Nehru family belonged to the saraswat Brahmin caste. Nehru graduated from Trinity College, Cambridge University and came back to India in 1912.

In 1916, by his parents' arrangement, he married seventeen-year-old Kamala.

He became the top political leader of the Indian National Congress Party along with his associate Mahatma Gandhi.

Nehru and his family followed Gandhi and abandoned fashionable British clothes and expensive possessions. Nehru and his family adopted the native language of Hindu or Hindustani for their common use.

Nehru used to wear a *khadi kurta* and a *Gandhi* cap as an Indian nationalist uniform. When Nehru's father joined the Swaraj Party in opposition to Gandhi, Jawaharlal Nehru did not join his father and stayed with Mahatma Gandhi. Together they led the nation of India to independence in 1947.

Nehru signed the first constitution of independent India in 1949. He was an outstanding public speaker.

Trivia

He was one of the founders of the international Non-Aligned Movement.

Quote

"A moment comes, which comes but rarely in history, when we step out from the old to the new; when an age ends; and when the soul of a nation long suppressed finds utterance."

JAYAPRAKASH NARAYAN

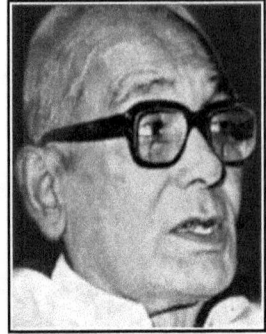

Popularly known as JP Narayan, Jayaprakash or Loknayak, Jayaprakash Narayan was born on October 11, 1902 in Sitabdiara, Saran in Bihar.

He was an Indian independence activist and political leader, remembered especially for leading the opposition to Indira Gandhi in the 1970s and for giving a call for peaceful Total Revolution.

J.P. Narayan was born in a Kayastha Family. His father Harsudayal was a junior official in the canal department of the State government and was often touring the region. Affectionately called *Baul*, Jayaprakash was left with his grandmother for studies.

His biography, *Jayaprakash*, was written by his nationalist friend and an eminent writer of Hindi literature, Ramavriksha Benipuri. He was posthumously awarded the **Bharat Ratna**, India's highest civilian award, in recognition of his social work in 1998.

He was also conferred with other awards including the 'Magsaysay Award' for Public Service in 1965. The airport of Patna is also named after him.

He died at the age of 79 on October 8, 1979 in Patna, Bihar.

Trivia

The then Prime Minister of India, Shri Charan Singh declared seven days mourning on the death of Shri J.P. Narayan calling him, 'the conscience of the nation'.

Quote

"If you really care for freedom, liberty, there cannot be any democracy or liberal institution without politics. The only true antidote to the perversions of politics is more politics and better politics. Not negation of politics."

📹 📹

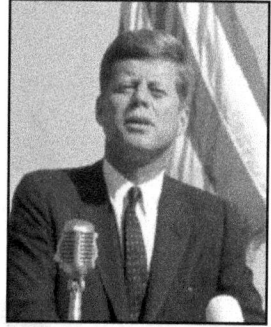

JOHN F KENNEDY

John Fitzgerald Kennedy with the nicknames like 'JFK', 'JACK' and "CRASH KENNEDY" was born on May 29, 1917 to Rose Kennedy and Joseph P Kennedy. John was named after his maternal grandfather, John 'HoneyFitz' Fitzgerald, the mayor of Boston. John kept on getting ill as a child and was given the last rites five times, the first one being when he was a newborn.

He was the second of four boys born to an Irish Catholic family with nine children: Joseph Jr., John, Robert F Kennedy (called Bobby), and Ted Kennedy (born Edward). Because Rose made Joe and Jack (the name his family called him) wear matching clothes, they fought a lot for attention.

John went to Choate, a private school. John went to Princeton, then Harvard, and for his senior thesis he wrote a piece about why England refused to get into the war until late. It was published in 1940 and called "Why England Slept".

John ran for Congress in Massachusetts in the early 1950's and won. He married Jacqueline Kennedy on September 12 1953. He became a father rather late in life. Their first child, Caroline Kennedy, was born on November 27, 1957 when John was 40 and their son, John Kennedy Jr., was born on November 25, 1960 when JFK was 43. They had a son named Patrick Bouvier, but he died a few days after birth.

On November 22, 1963, John was to give a speech in Dallas, but on his way an assassin hidden on the sixth floor of the Texas School Book Depository opened fire at Kennedy, who was riding in an open car. Hit twice and severely wounded, Kennedy died in a local hospital at 1:00 pm. Lee Harvey Oswald, the assassin was captured after a short period of time for interrogation.

Trivia

He was the youngest elected US President.

Quote

"Ask not what your country can do for you; ask what you can do for your country."

65

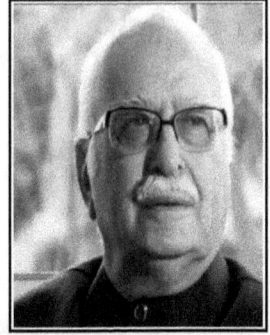

L.K. ADVANI

Lal Kishanchand Advani, popularly known as Lal Krishna Advani or L.K. Advani, was born on November 8, 1927 in Karachi, Pakistan (then, British India). He is a veteran Indian politician and a former president of the Bharatiya Janata Party (BJP). The BJP is currently the major opposition party in the country.

L.K. Advani has served as the Deputy Prime Minister of India from 2002 to 2004 and was the Leader of the Opposition in the tenth and the 14th Lok Sabha.

Advani began his political career as a worker of the Rashtriya Swayamsevak Sangh (RSS) and is often credited with having made the BJP an alarming force in Indian politics. He was elected as the Secretary of the RSS in 1947.

Advani has seen the formation of the BJP – from Jana Sangh to Janata Party and then the Bharatiya Janata Party. The unpopularity of the emergency called by the then Prime Minister Indira Gandhi in 1975 helped the BJP to get a landslide victory. Adavni served as the Minister of Information and Broadcasting in the Morarji Desai government.

In the 1990s, Advani took the party to new heights. BJP became the single largest party, thus forming the government with Atal Bihari Vajpayee as its Prime Minister in 1996. However, Vajpayee resigned after 13 days. The BJP again came into power under the umbrella of 'National Democratic Alliance' in 1998. He was also projected as Prime Ministerial candidate in 2009 elections.

The Congress emerged victorious in 2009 general elections while the BJP holds position of the main opposition. Mr. L.K. Advani has taken six major *yatras* throughout India, like the *Ram Rath Yatra, Janadesh Yatra, Swarna Jayanti Rath Yatra, Uday Yatra and Jan Chetna Yatra*. The most recent one is the *Jan Chetna Yatra* against corruption.

Trivia

He is married to Kamla Advani and has two children, Pratibha and Jayant.

📹 📹

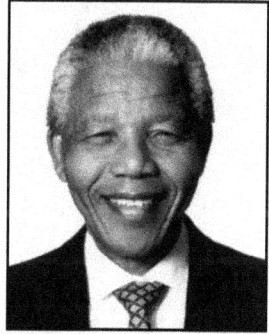

NELSON MANDELA

Nelson Mandela alias Rolihlahla was born on the July 18, 1918 in a small village of Mvezo, in Umtata, South Africa. He became actively involved in the Anti-apartheid Movement and joined the African National Congress (ANC) in 1942.

He directed a campaign of peaceful, non-violent defiance against the South African government and its racist policies for 20 years.

Following the suggestion of one of Rolihlahla's father's friends, he was baptised into the Methodist Church and became the first in his family to attend school. As was the custom at the time and probably due to the bias of the British educational system in South Africa, his teacher told him that his new first name would be ' elson'.

Nelson Mandela is known as the leader of the African National Congress (ANC) and for his lifelong struggle against Apartheid (enforced racial separation), which was instituted in South Africa in 1948. The ANC was soon declared a terrorist organisation and banned by the South African government.

Mandela was arrested in 1962 and imprisoned for life on 'terrorist' charges, but in 1990, he was freed by South African President FW de Klerk. In 1994, he was elected President of South Africa. Two biographical movies were made, and the latest, *Mandela and de Klerk* (1997), focused on his life's struggles. He died on April 1, 2010 at Cape Town, South Africa.

Trivia

He was first Black President of the Republic of South Africa from 1994 to 1999.

Quote

"A good head and a good heart are always a formidable combination."

RONALD REAGAN

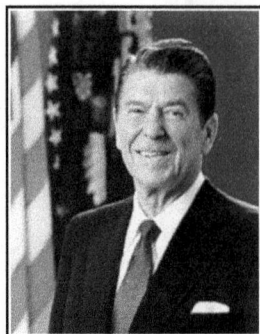

Ronald Reagan was born on February 6, 1911 in Illinois. He was the 40th President of the United States.

Reagan worked as a radio sports announcer for WOC radio in Davenport after graduating from the Eureka College in 1932. Before entering politics, Reagan was an actor. His started when his acting career he was asked to play a radio announcer in 'Love is on the air' in 1937.

Reagan became a famous actor by the time he did his last film, 'The Killers' in 1964.

He married actress Jane Wyman in 1940. The couple got divorced in 1948 during the time when Reagan was becoming politically active. Then, in 1952, he married actress Nancy Davis. The couple had two children.

Reagan switched political parties after actively supporting Nixon's campaign for President in 1960 and officially became a Republican in 1962.

In 1966, Reagan successfully ran for the 'Governor of California' and served two consecutive terms. He then won the Presidential elections for the United States in 1980.

He made the first major move forward in the Cold War when he and Russian leader Mikhail Gorbachev agreed to jointly eliminate some of their nuclear weapons.

After serving two consecutive terms as President, Reagan retired. He was soon officially diagnosed with Alzheimer's disease and decided to tell the American people in an open letter on November 5, 1994.

Reagan's health continued to deteriorate and on June 5, 2004, Reagan passed away at the age of 93.

Trivia

Republican Ronald Reagan became the 'oldest President elected' when he took office as the 40th President of the United States.

SAMUEL ADAMS

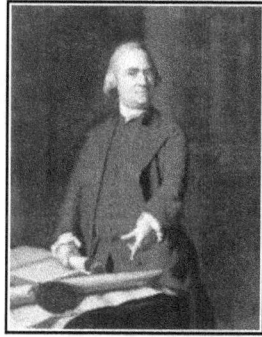

Samuel Adams was born on September 27, 1722. He was an American statesman, political philosopher and one of the Founding Fathers of the United States. As a politician in colonial Massachusetts, Adams was a leader of the movement that became the American Revolution, and was one of the architects of the principles of American republicanism that shaped the political culture of the United States. He was a second cousin to President John Adams.

A graduate of Harvard College, he was an unsuccessful businessman and tax collector before concentrating on politics.

After Parliament passed the 'Coercive Acts' in 1774, Adams attended the Continental Congress in Philadelphia, which was convened to coordinate a colonial response. He helped to guide the Congress towards issuing the Declaration of Independence in 1776, and helped draft the Articles of Confederation and the Massachusetts Constitution. Adams returned to Massachusetts after the American Revolution, where he served in the state senate and was eventually elected the governor.

Samuel Adams is a controversial figure in American history. Accounts written in the 19th century praised him as someone who had been steering his fellow colonists towards independence long before the outbreak of the Revolutionary War. This view gave way to negative assessments of Adams in the first half of the 20th century, in which he was portrayed as a master of propaganda who provoked mob violence to achieve his goals. Both of these interpretations have been challenged by some modern scholars, who argue that these traditional depictions of Adams are myths contradicted by the historical record.

Trivia
The younger Samuel Adams attended the Boston Latin School.

Quote
"How strangely will the Tools of a Tyrant pervert the plain Meaning of Words!"

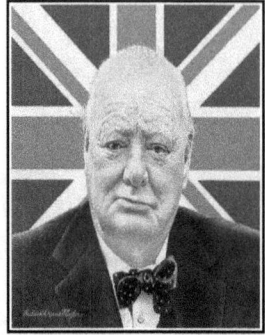

WINSTON CHURCHILL

Popularly known by the name 'Winnie' and 'The British Bulldog', Winston Churchill was born in Blenheim Palace, England. His mother's name was Lady Randolph Churchill who had American lineage. He was the grandson of the seventh Duke of Marlborough from his father's side.

After completing his education from famous English public schools, such as Harrow, he went on to fulfil his ambition for a life in the army. He fought in various parts of the British Empire until in 1900 when he won the Conservative seat in Oldham in the general election. From here until 1929, he held various offices in the British arliament.

Winston Churchill, the First Lord of the Admiralty, was chosen to become Prime Minister at the age of 65. It could be said that Churchill's fiery energy had never been experienced before in British politics and suddenly, it seemed as though Britain could face the Nazi giant.

He was re-elected as Prime Minister in 1951 but because of deteriorating health, he left the public scene. He died at Hyde Park Gate, London, on January 24, 1965 at the age of 90. His daughter Mary wrote to him on his deathbed. 'I owe you what every Englishman, woman and child owes you – liberty itself'.

Trivia
He is buried in a modest churchyard in Bladon, not far from his birthplace at Blenheim Palace. Chartwell, his countryhouse, is open to the public. Much of his paintings were done there.

Quote
"History will be kind to me for I intend to write it."

📹 📹

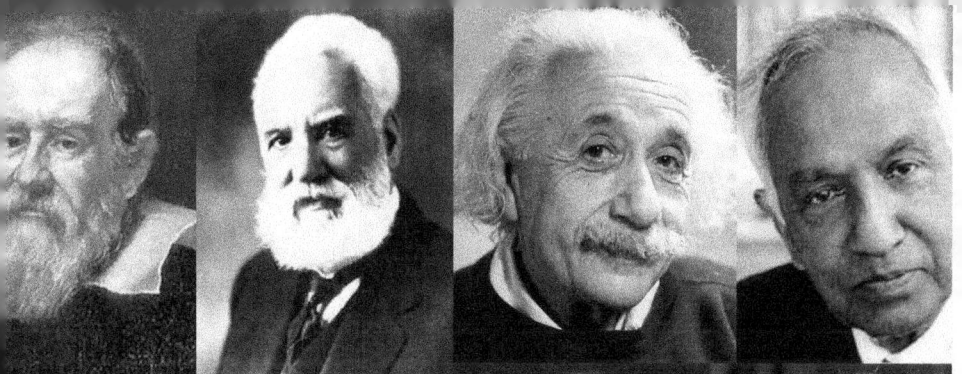

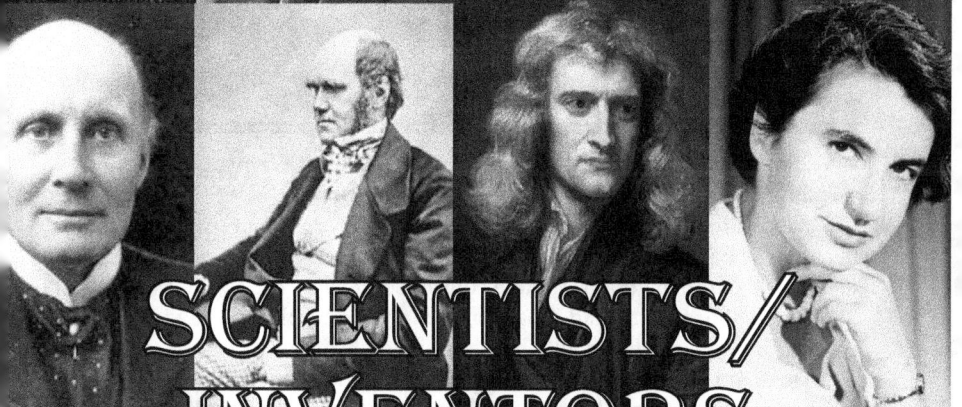

SCIENTISTS/INVENTORS

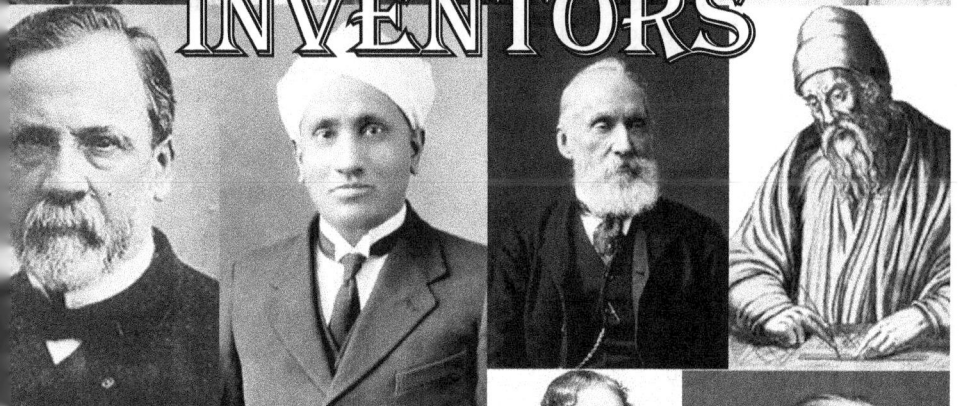

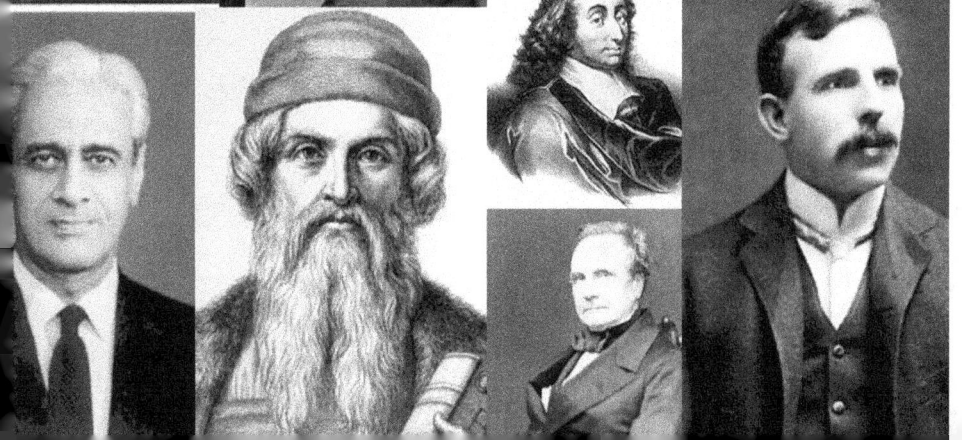

ALBERT EINSTEIN

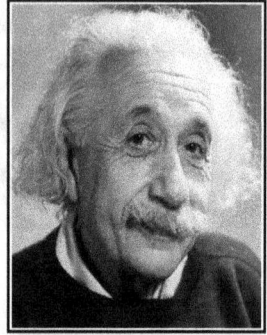

Albert Einstein was born on March 14, 1879 in Ulm, Germany. As a child, he was always fascinated by science and its powers.

Known to the world as a genius, Einstein has carried out researches that became the basis for many equipments that we use on a day to day basis, like television, automatic doors, remote controlled devices, etc.

As a child, he also had a passion for music and played the violin and piano. This passion stayed with him even when he grew up.

He spent his childhood moving from Germany to Italy and later to Switzerland from where he graduated from the High School in 1896.

In 1905, he worked as a patent clerk in Bern, Switzerland. It was then that he published four of his most popular research papers and earned his doctoral degree. These papers included his Special Theory of Relativity and his famous equation $E=mc^2$.

Later in 1915, he came up with his *General Theory of Relativity*. He received the **Nobel Prize in Physics** in 1921 for it.

In 1933, he moved to the United States and became a professor at the Institute of Advanced Study in Princeton, New Jersey.

Einstein's researches and important works include Relativity, Special Theory of Relativity, General Theory of Relativity, Investigations on Theory of Brownian Movement and The Evolution of Physics.

Among his non-scientific works include: About Zionism, Why War?, My Philosophy and Out of My Later Years are the most popular.

Trivia
Albert Einstein could not speak fluently until the age of nine.

Quote
"A person who never made a mistake never tried anything new."

ALEXANDER GRAHAM BELL

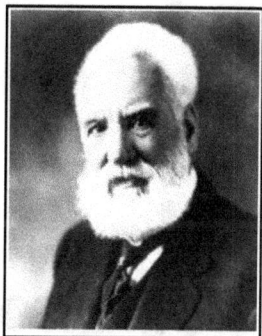

Born in Edinburgh, Scotland on March 3, 1847, Alexander Graham Bell was an inventor and a scientist. His father was Alexander Melville Bell, who was a leading authority in speech correction. Bell was mainly educated at home. However, he spent two years in Edinburgh Royal High School and also attended a few lectures at the Edinburgh University.

Bell began his career in 1864 as a teacher at the Elgin's Western House Academy. Later, he moved to London and became his father's assistant. Like his other brothers, who died of tuberculosis, Bell's health began to deteriorate. The family decided to move to Canada in 1870. Soon after they settled in Southern Ontario, Bell's health began to improve.

Bell gave lectures on visible speech, which is a method of teaching speech to the deaf. He was invited to give a series of speeches in the United States in 1871. He then opened a school for teachers of the deaf in Boston and in 1873 became professor of vocal physiology at the city's university.

He has the credit of giving the *first telephone* to the world. After a series of experiments with several acoustical devices, Bell produced the first intelligible telephonic transmission with a message to his assistant, Thomas Watson, on June 5, 1875. Bell patented his telephone on March 3, 1876 after he came to know that electrical engineer, Elisha Gray was also working on a similar project. He formed the Bell Telephone Company in 1877. The telephone was an instant success.

Trivia

His invention of telephone was widely accepted and within three years, there were around 30,000 telephones in use around the world. Elisha Gray later claimed the invention of the telephone but lost the long legal battle in the Supreme Court.

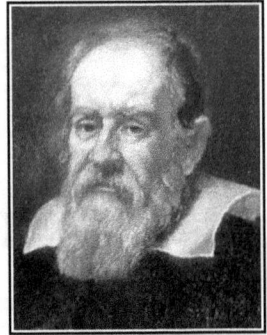

GALILEO GALILEI

Italian physicist, mathematician, astronomer, and philosopher, Galileo Galilei was born on February 15, 1564.

He is often refered to as the 'Father of Modern Observational Astronomy', 'Father of Modern Physics' and the 'Father of Modern Science'.

Commonly known as 'Galileo', he played a major role in the Scientific Revolution.

His achievements include improvements to the telescope and consequent astronomical observations in addition to the support for Copernicanism. According to physicist Stephen Hawking, Galileo Galilei was responsible for the birth of modern science.

Galileo's major contributions to observational astronomy include the telescopic confirmation of the phases of Venus, the observation and analysis of sunspots and the discovery of the four largest satellites of Jupiter. The satellites are named after him as the *Galilean moons* in his honour.

Galileo also worked in applied science and technology, inventing an improved military compass and other instruments.

He died after he suffered fever and heart palpitations in 1642 at the age of 77.

Galileo's heliocentrism was controversial within his lifetime, when most subscribed to either Geocentrism or the Tychonic system. He was opposed by astronomers, who doubted his theory due to the absence of an observed stellar parallax.

After investigations by the Roman Inquisition in 1615, they concluded that it could only be supported as a possibility, not as an established fact. Galileo was tried and was put under house arrest. It was during this time that he wrote one of his finest works, *Two New Sciences.*

Trivia

Three of Galileo's fingers and a tooth were removed from his mortal remains, while he was being reburied in the main body of basilica at a monument constructed in his honour. The middle finger is currently on exhibition at the Muse Galileo in Italy.

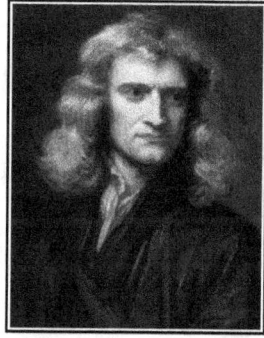

ISAAC NEWTON

I saac Newton was born on December 25, 1642. He was an English physicist, mathematician, astronomer, natural philosopher, alchemist, and theologian and has been "considered by many to be the greatest and most influential scientist, who ever lived. He was most famous for his three laws of *motion*, but was also known for other major discoveries in maths and science.

He compiled most of his works into a masterpiece of science called the *Principia*. Newton was known to be arrogant, so his book was written almost exclusively for the elite and the rich.

Some people claim that only 50 people in history have been able to understand his style of writing. Despite his arrogance, he truly was a father in the field of science. At the age of 18, he had devised a new system of mathematics called the *Calculus*.

He developed three laws which resulted in a new way of understanding motion. All of this happened at his farm while the Black Plague swept across England. In the *Principia*, Newton claimed to have "discovered" gravity when an apple fell on his head. But, many now believe that this was just a story told by Newton, and that in real life, he discovered gravity through thinking a not seeing.

He died on March 20, 1727 at Kensington, England.

Trivia

'Newton's Gravitational Theory' was not inspired by a Falling Apple.

Quote

"This most beautiful system, [The Universe] could only proceed from the dominion of an intelligent and powerful Being."

JOHANNES GUTENBERG

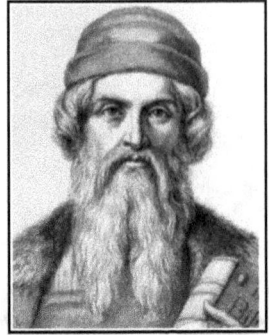

Born in 1398, Johannes Gutenberg was a German inventor of a method of printing from the movable type.

He started experimenting with printing by 1438. In 1440, Gutenberg invented a *printing press* process that remained the principal means of printing until the late 20th century.

His method of printing from movable type allowed, for the first time, the mass production of printed books. It also included the use of metal moulds and alloys, a special press and oil-based inks.

Gutenberg's printing technology rapidly spread across Europe and quickly replaced most of the handwritten manuscript methods of book production throughout the world.

'Woodblock printing', 'engraving' and 'rubrication' continued to be used to supplement Gutenberg's printing process.

His first major work using his printing methods was the *Gutenberg Bible* between 1450 and 1455.

The entire *Gutenberg Bible* is likely to fetch an estimated 100 million dollars if it is made available on the world market. An original individual leaf can fetch around $100,000.

Gutenberg's work is material in the world. Johann Gutenberg died in Mainz, Germany on 1468. The inventor could not make profits from his inventions and died in poverty.

Trivia

His full name was Johannes Gensfleisch zur Laden zum Gutenberg.

🎥 🎥

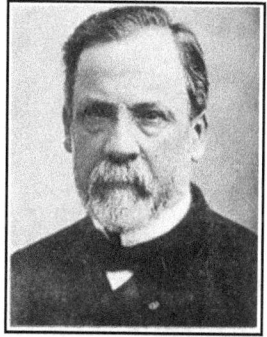

LOUIS PASTEUR

Born on December 27, 1822, Louis Pasteur was a French chemist and microbiologist. Remembered for his remarkable breakthroughs in the causes and preventions of diseases, his discoveries reduced mortality from puerperal fever.

He created the *first vaccine* for rabies and anthrax. His experiments supported the *germ theory of disease.*

Best known to people for inventing the process called *pasteurisation,* he is regarded as one of the three main founders of microbiology, together with Ferdinand Cohn and Robert Koch.

Louis grew up in the town of Arbois and gained degrees in Mathematical Sciences before entering an elite college, École Normale Supérieure.

After serving briefly as a professor of physics at Dijon Lycée in 1848, he became the professor of chemistry at the University of Strasbourg. At the University of Strasbourg, he met and courted Marie Laurent in 1849. They were married on May 29, 1849. The couple had five children. Out of his five children, only two survived till adulthood, the other three died of typhoid. These tragedies inspired Pasteur to try to find cures for diseases, such as *typhoid.*

Pasteur also made many discoveries in the field of chemistry, the most notable one being the molecular basis for the asymmetry of certain crystals.

He died on September 28, 1895. His body lies beneath the Institute Pasteur in Paris in a spectacular vault cover.

Trivia

In 1995, the centennial of the death of Louis Pasteur, the New York Times ran an article titled, 'Pasteur's Deception'. After reading Pasteur's lab notes thoroughly, the science historian, Gerald L Geison declared that Pasteur had given a misleading account of the preparation of the anthrax vaccine used in the experiment at Pouilly-le-Fort.

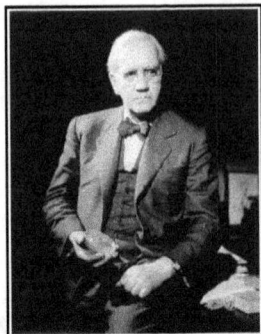

SIR ALEXANDER FLEMING

Sir Alexander Fleming was born on August 6, 1881 at Lochfield, Scotland. He was a Scottish biologist and pharmacologist.

He wrote many articles on bacteriology, immunology and chemotherapy.

His best-known discoveries are the discovery of the enzyme, *lysozyme* in 1923 and the antibiotic substance, penicillin from the mould, *Penicillium notatum* in 1928. He shared the **Nobel Prize in Physiology or Medicine** in 1945 with Howard Florey and Ernst Boris Chain.

The active ingredient Penicillin in the *Penicillium notatum* turned out to be an infection-fighting agent of enormous potenc .

It was the most efficacious life-saving drug in the world. Penicillin could alter the treatment of bacterial infections forever. By the middle of the century, Fleming's discovery had spawned a hug pharmaceutical industry churning out synthetic penicillin that would conquer some of mankind's most ancient scourges.

In 1955, Fleming died at his home in London of a heart attack. He was buried at St Paul's Cathedral.

Trivia

The Time magazine named Fleming one of the 100 Most Important People of the 20th Century for his discovery of penicillin in 1999.

Quote

"I have been trying to point out that in our lives, chance may have an astonishing influence and, if I may offer advice to the young laboratory worker, it would be this – never to neglect an extraordinary appearance or happening."

THE WRIGHT BROTHERS

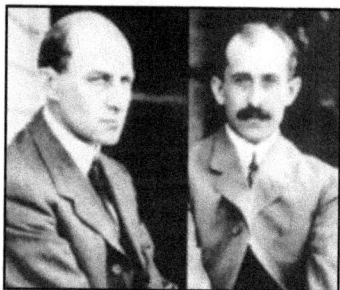

The Wright Brothers, **Wilbur** and **Orville Wright,** Perhaps the most influential brothers in history, were the sons of a bishop of the United Brethren in Christ Milton Wright.

Wilbur was born on April 16, 1867 in Millville, Indiana, while Orville was born on August 19, 1871 in Dayton, Ohio.

The two were inseparable until the death of Wilbur in 1912. Their personalities were perfectly complementary to each other providing what the other lacked. While, Orville was full of ideas and enthusiasm, Wilbur was more mature in his judgements and more likely to see a project through.

In their early years, Orville and Wilbur helped their father, who edited a journal called the 'Religious Telescope'. Later, they began a publication of a four-page weekly newspaper, 'West Side News'.

In 1829, they started a bicycle repair shop and a factory, and started making aerial experiments with kites and gliders in 1896.

After having failed many flight experiments, the Wrights thought that it would be better to control a plane by moving its wings.

In 1900, they made their first flight to Kitty Hawk, North Carolina and set up a camp there. They confirmed their data by making thousands of flights in two years and then were determined to apply power to their machine.

Soon, they made a 12 horsepower engine, weighing 750 pounds. It proved to be capable of travelling 31 miles per hour.

Both of them made many record-breaking flights near Le Mans and France. Wilbur died on May 30, 1912 and Orville died on January 30, 1948.

Trivia

Orville lived quietly in Dayton after Wilbur's death, conducting experiments on mechanical problems of interest to him.

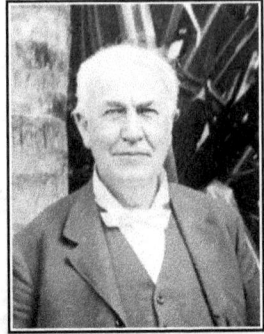

THOMAS EDISON

Thomas Edison was born on February 11, 1847 in Milan, US. Born in a small town in the Midwest, in Ohio, young Thomas was a restless student whose mind often wondered as the teacher gave lessons. But, it was his mother that would educate him at home.

He invented *the phonograph, the incandescent electric lightbulb, the alkaline storage battery* among other things. He held more than 900 patents and laid the foundation for the 'modern electric age'.

It would not be until Thomas Edison and his new wife moved to New Jersey that his career would really unfold. There, he unveiled his automatic repeater that would revolutionise the telegraph world. He also displayed his *phonograph*, the first device of its kind to record and play back sound. The invention so frightened the crowd that they believed him to be a sorcerer. With better design and longer-lasting records, the phonograph became a huge hit at home and abroad – especially in England.

He went on to form the 'Edison Electric Light Company' in New York City. The small company provided the first lights to lower Manhattan, New York. Thomas Edison's dream was to provide every American household with affordable electric power. He continued working on his inventions, even designing phone speakers that were used through the latter 20th century.

He died on 18th October 1931, West Orange, New Jersey, USA with complications of diabetes.

Trivia
He was a member of the Academy of Motion Picture Arts & Sciences (AMPAS).

Quote
"Anything that won't sell, I don't want to invent. Its sale is proof of utility, and utility is success."

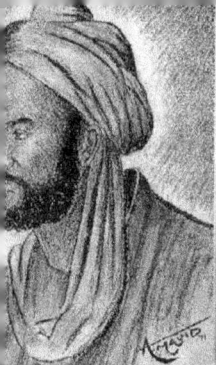

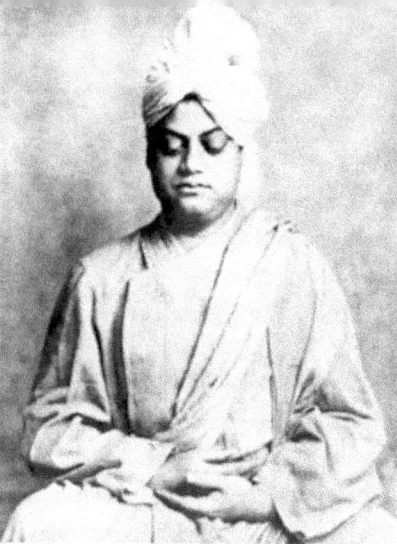

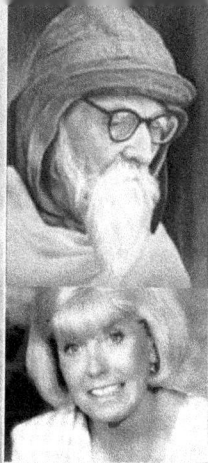

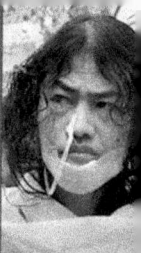

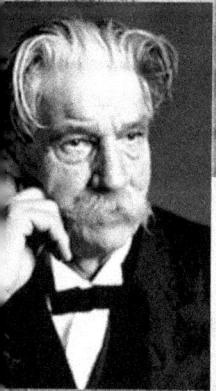

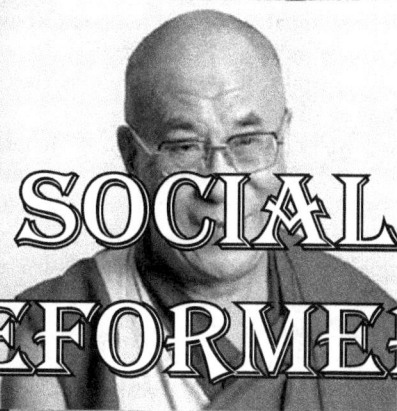

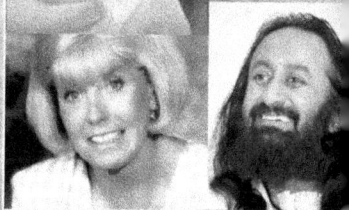

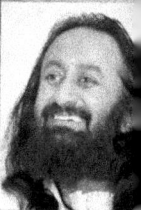

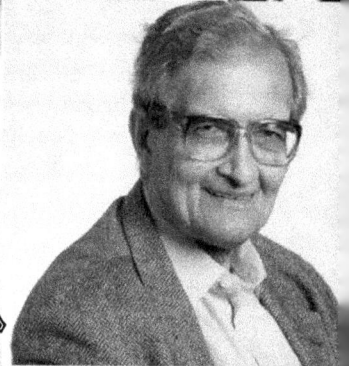

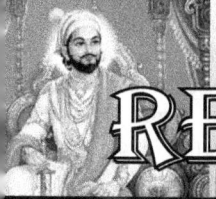

SOCIAL REFORMERS

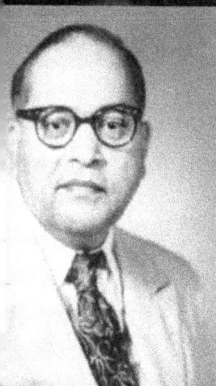

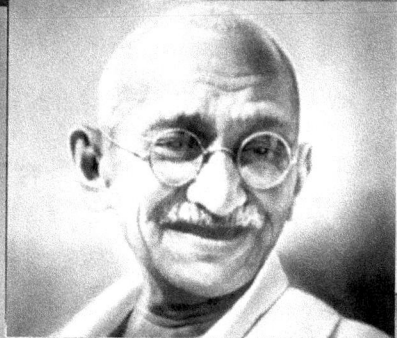

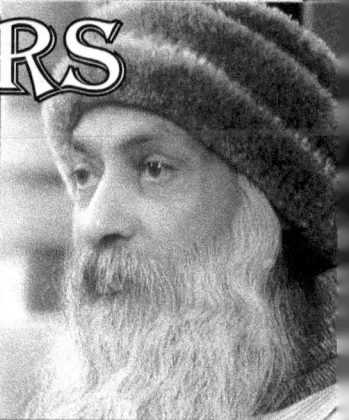

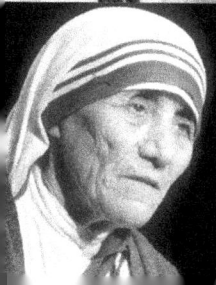

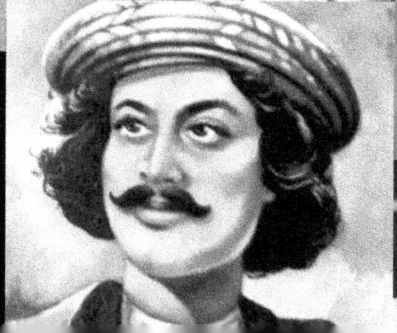

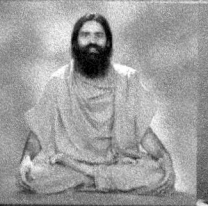

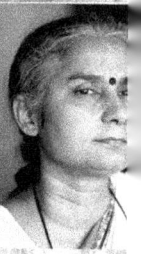

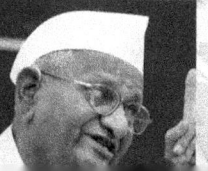

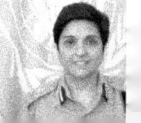

ACHARYA VINOBA BHAVE

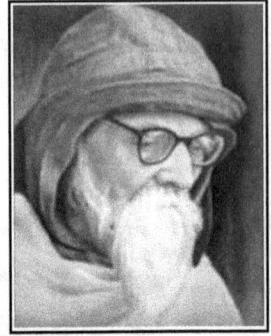

Born on September 11, 1895, Acharya Vinoba Bhave was considered as Mahatma Gandhi's spiritual successor. Vinobha Bhave's original name was Vinayak Narahari Bhave and was born in a Brahmin family in Maharashtra.

His 'Bhoodan' (Gift of the Land) Movement started on April 18, 1951 and attracted the attention of the world.

Vinoba Bhave was well-read in the writings of Maharashtra's saints and philosophers and was also deeply interested in Mathematics.

In 1916, while he was on his way to Mumbai to appear for the intermediate examination, he took a detour and reached Varanasi. He was motivated by his desire to attain the imperishable. He studied ancient Sanskrit texts in Varanasi.

After exchange of few letters between Bhave and Mahatma Gandhi, Vinoba Bhave went and met Gandhiji on June 7, 1916 which changed the course of Bhave's life. He developed a deep bond with Gandhiji and participated in the activities at Gandhi's ashram with keen interest.

Vinoba Bhave was asked by Gandhiji to take charge of the ashram at Wardha in 1921. In 1923, he brought out the *Maharashtra Dharma*, a monthly in Marathi, which had his essays on the Upanishads.

In 1940, Bhave was chosen by Gandhi to be the first Individual *Satyagrahi*. Vinoba Bhave also participated in the 'Quit India Movement'.

After independence, he started the social reform movements, such as Bhoodan Movement and Sarvodaya Movement.

He died on November 15, 1982 after refusing food and medicine few days earlier. He was *posthumously* honoured with the **Bharat Ratna** in 1984.

Trivia

He observed a *year of silence* from December 25, 1974 to December 25, 1975 and in 1976, undertook a fast to stop the slaughter of cows.

📽️ 📽️

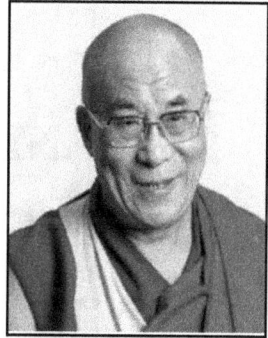

Dalai Lama

His holiness, the 14th Dalai Lama, born as Tenzin Gyatso, is Tibet's head of state as well as the spiritual leader of the Tibetan people.

The Dalai Lama was born in Taktser, Qinghai, and was selected as the rebirth of the 13th Dalai Lama, two years later, although he was only formally recognised as the 14th on the November 17, 1950, at the age of 15.

He inherited control over a government controlling area roughly corresponding to the Tibet Autonomous Region just as the nascent People's Republic of China wished to reassert central control over it. There is a dispute over whether the respective governments reached an agreement for a joint Communist-Lamaist administration.

His Holiness assumed full power of Tibet in November 1950. He completed his 'Doctorate of Buddhist Philosophy' in 1959, the same year when China attacked Tibet, after which he escaped to Dharamsala, India, from where he has since then led the Tibetan government in exile.

On December 10, 1989, His Holiness accepted the Nobel Peace Prize *'on behalf of the oppressed everywhere and all those, who struggle for freedom and work for world peace and the people of Tibet'.* In his acceptance statement, he declared, 'This prize reaffirms our conviction that with truth, courage, and determination as our weapons, Tibet will be liberated. Our struggle must remain non-violent and free of hatred'.

Trivia

Tenzin was awarded the Christmas Humphreys Award from the Buddhist Society of the United Kingdom on May 28, 2004.

Quote

"Be kind whenever possible. It is always possible."

MOHANDAS KARAMCHAND GANDHI

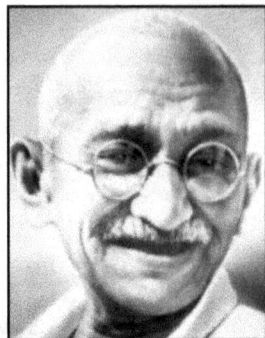

Mohandas Karamchand Gandhi (October 2, 1869 – January 30, 1948) was the pre-eminent political and ideological leader of India during the Indian Independence Movement.

A pioneer of *satyagraha*, or resistance to tyranny through Mass Civil Disobedience – a philosophy firmly founded upon *ahimsa*, or total non-violence – Gandhi led India to independence and inspired movements for civil rights and freedom across the world.

Gandhi is often referred to as the *Mahatma* or the "Great Soul," an honorific first applied to him by Rabindranath Tagore. In India, he is also called *Bapu* and officially honoured as the **Father of the Nation**. His birthday, October 2, is commemorated in India as *Gandhi Jayanti*, a national holiday, and worldwide as the 'International Day of Non-Violence'.

Gandhi first employed non-violent civil disobedience as an expatriate lawyer in South Africa, in the resident Indian community's struggle for civil rights.

After his return to India in 1915, he set about organising peasants, farmers, and urban labourers in protesting excessive land-tax and discrimination. Assuming leadership of the Indian National Congress in 1921, Gandhi led nationwide campaigns for easing poverty, expanding women's rights, building religious and ethnic amity, ending untouchability, increasing economic self-reliance, but above all for achieving *Swaraj* – the independence of India from foreign domination. Gandhi famously led Indians in protesting the British-imposed salt tax with the 400 km (250 miles) *Dandi Salt March* in 1930, and later in calling for the British to 'Quit India' in 1942.

Trivia

He was imprisoned for many years, on many occasions, in both South Africa and India.

🎥 🎥

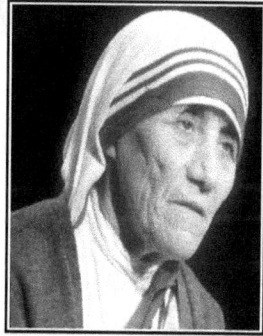

MOTHER TERESA

The image of a short woman in a white sari with blue border with kindness in her eyes and the will to help in her heart, reminds of Mother Teresa (August 26, 1910 – September 5, 1997).

Born in Skopje, the Republic of Macedonia, to well-to-do parents, Mother Teresa always knew in her heart that she was born to serve the poor. At the age of 18, she was given permission to join a group of nuns in Ireland. After a few months of training in Dublin, she travelled to Kolkata, accepted the vows of a nun, and took the name, Teresa.

Touched by the poverty around her in Calcutta (Kolkata), while teaching at St. Mary's High School for Girls, she left the school and started working in the slums of Calcutta and opened an open-air school for children. Soon, many volunteers joined her and many funded the good cause. She soon started 'The Missionaries of Charity'.

Today, the institution has many well trained doctors, nurses and social workers working to help the poor and the victims of natural catastrophes like floods, famine, epidemics, etc. It has also got many branches worldwide. In a time, when leprosy stricken people were a common sight around Calcutta, and people wouldn't even look at the lepers, Mother Teresa hugged them, changed their bandages, and took care of them.

She also started a *lepers' colony* called 'Shanti'. She was awarded the **Nobel Peace Prize** for her sacrificial work towards those in need

Trivia

Mother Teresa's real name was Agnes Gonxha Bojaxhiu. Agnes Bojaxhiu was her family name and Gonxha, her middle name. Gonxha means 'flower bud' in Albania and people often called her by this name.

Quote

"Being unwanted, unloved, uncared for, forgotten by everybody, I think that is a much greater hunger, a much greater poverty than the person who has nothing to eat."

Raja Ram Mohan Roy

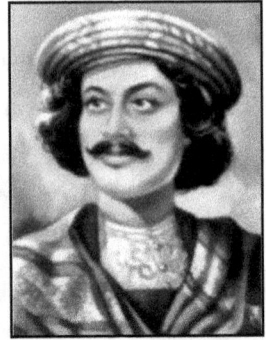

Born in a famous family of Bengal in 1772, Raja Ram Mohan Roy was a great scholar of Sanskrit, Persian and English and knew Arabic, Latin and Greek.

He was one of the greatest social reformers that India has produced. He was instrumental in eradicating social evils like *Sati, Purdah* and *Child Marriage* from the Indian soil and therefore, rightly called the 'Father of Modern India'.

He also advocated equal rights of widows to remarry, rights for women, and right of women to property but his fight to eradicate Sati is a landmark in Indian history.

Having a rational and scientific approach, he believed in the principle of human dignity and social equality. He read the Hindu scriptures and other books of other religions.

He joined the service of the East India Company in 1805 and gradually rose to high offices

He, along with Dwarkanath Tagore and others, founded the Brahmo Sabha in 1828, which engendered the Brahmo Samaj, which was an influential Indian socio-religious reform movement during the "Bengal Renaissance".

Roy wrote a book in Persian the 'Gift of Monotheists' in 1809. He preached that 'God in one' and believed in universal brotherhood. In one of his books, 'Precepts of Jesus', published in 1820, he tried to clear the difference between the moral and philosophic message of the 'New Testament'.

Raja Ram Mohan Roy died at Bristol in England in 1833 due to meningitis.

Trivia

Roy married thrice in his lifetime. His third wife, Uma devi outlived him. Mughal emperor Akbar shah II conferred on him the title of 'Raja'.

SWAMI VIVEKANANDA

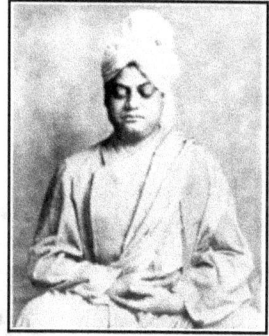

Swami Vivekananda was born to Viswanath Dutta and Bhuvaneswari Devi on January 12, 1863 in Shimla Pally of Kolkata, West Bengal. This precocious child started meditating at a very early age. Even as a child, he was an all rounder. One of the most inspiring personalities of India, who did a lot to make India a better place to live in, within a short span of time, Vivekananda achieved a lot and went a long way in serving humans. He was the principal disciple of Sri Ramakrishna Paramahamsa.

The *Ramakrishna Mission* was founded by Swami Vivekananda, on the 1st of May in the year 1897. The Ramakrishna Mission is actively involved in the missionary as well as altruistic works, such as disaster relief. The disciples that are serving the mission consist of both monastic and householder. Its headquarters are based near Kolkata, India.

He compiled a number of books on the four Yogas, namely the *Raja Yoga, Karma Yoga, Bhakti Yoga* and the *Jnana Yoga*. His best works include the letters written by him. He maintained a very simple style of writing, so that the laymen, are able to understand his each and every word. He was not just actively involved in writing, but also was a great singer and composed several songs.

On July 4, 1902, at a young age of 39, this great man headed his way for heaven.

Trivia

Before turning into a monastic, Vivekananda was called by the name Narendranath Dutta.

SPORTSPERSONS

ANDRE AGASSI

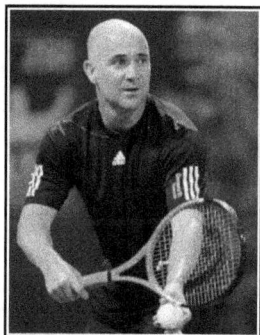

A ndre Kirk Agassi was born on April 29, 1970 in Las Vegas to Emmanuel Mike Aghassian and Betty. He is a retired American professional tennis player. At the age of 13, he went to Nick Bollettieri's Tennis Academy in Florida, where he was coached for free. He had a natural talent for the game.

Agassi turned professional at the age of 16. By the end of the year, he was ranked no 91. In 1987, he won the singles title in the Sul American Open in Itaparica and ended ranked world no 25. After winning several tournaments in 1988, his year end ranking was world No 3. The Association of Tennis Professionals and the Tennis Magazine named him as the Most Improved Player of the Year, 1988.

He reached his first Grand Slam Final in 1990 at the French Open. In the same year, Agassi won the *Davis Cup*, a victory for America after eight years, and won his only Tennis Masters Cup. He played in Wimbledon in 1991. He won the 'Wimbledon' title in 1992 and was the BBC Overseas Sports Personality of the Year.

Agassi won the Australian Open in 1995, the first appearance in the event. He reached the world no 1 ranking in April 1995. At the Olympic Games, Agassi won the men's singles gold medal in Atlanta. In 1999, he became only the fifth male player to have won all four grand slam titles during his career. He was also the first male player in history to have won all four grand slam titles on three different surfaces. Agassi was also the first male player to win the Career Golden Slam.

In 2006, while in Wimbledon Agassi announced his retirement. He has earned more US$ 30 million in his career and more than US$ 25 million a year in endorsements.

Agassi married actress Brooke Shields on April 19, 1997 and the couple filed for divorce less than two years later. Agassi and Steffi Graf married in 2001. They have two children and live in Las Vegas area. In 2005, the Tennis magazine named him the seventh greatest male player and the 12th greatest player overall for the period, 1965 through 2005. In 2011, Agassi was inducted into the International Tennis Hall of Fame at a ceremony in Newport, Rhode Island.

DIEGO MARADONA

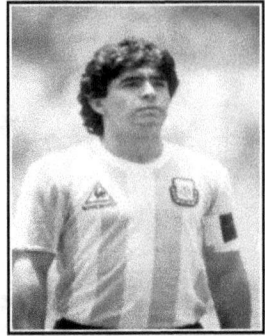

Diego Armando Maradona was born on October 30, 1960. He is a retired Argentine football player. He was born in Lanus and raised in Villa Fiorito near Buenos Aires. Maradona was playing in his neighbourhood club at the age of ten when he was spotted by a talent scout. He played for the Los Cebollitas, junior team of Buenos Aires.

Maradona made his professional debut in 1976 with Argentinos Juniors. He was transferred to the Boca Juniors in 1981. In 1982, he was transferred to Barcelona in Spain after the 1982 World Cup. Barcelona won the 'Copa Del Ray' in 1983. He was then transferred to Napoli in 1984.

Led by Maradona, Napoli reached its most successful era in its history. They won Serie A Italian Championships, Coppa Italia in 1987, the UEFA Cup in 1989 and the Italian Super Cup in 1990. He was banned for 15 months after failing a drug test for cocaine and left Napoli.

Maradona's first World Cup was in 1982. He captained the Argentine national team to victory in the 1986 World Cup. During the quarter final against England his second goal was voted by FIFA as the greatest goal in the history of World Cup. The goal was voted Goal of the Century in 2002 online poll conducted by FIFA. In a tribute to Maradona, the Azteca Stadium authorities built a statue of him scoring the Goal of the Century and placed it at the entrance of the stadium.

In 1990, Argentina reached the finals but lost to West Germany. Maradona published his autobiography, 'Yo Soy El Diego' (I am The Diego). In 2000, Maradona finished top of the poll conducted by FIFA, making him the 'Player of the Century'. Maradona has also won polls for Best Goal Ever Scored in a World Cup and All-Time Ultimate World Cup Team. The Argentine Juniors named their stadium after Maradona in 2003.

Maradona became the host of a talk-variety show on Argentine television, *La Noche del 10* ("The Night of the Number 10) in 2005.

Serbian filmmaker, Emir Kusturica made a documentary, *Maradona* on the player's life. Maradona was appointed the 'Goodwill Ambassador' of IIMSAM. In 2010, Maradona was chosen No. 1 in the Greatest 10 World Cup players of all time by the *Times*, a London based paper.

Kapil Dev

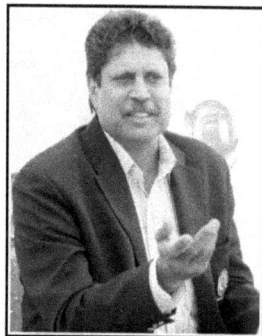

Kapil Dev Ramlal Nikhanj better known as Kapil Dev is a former Indian cricketer and said to be one of the all time greatest all-rounders to have existed in the world of Cricket.

Born on January 6, 1959 in Chandigarh, Kapil Dev began his Cricket career in Domestic Cricket from the Haryana team, with a match played against Punjab team in November 1975.

Kapil gave best performance of his initial times in a match against Bengal, in which he took seven wickets giving only 20 runs within nine overs in the second innings.

He debuted in the Test Cricket in 1978 against Pakistan and played his first One-Day International (DI) on October 1, 1978 against Pakistan.

Kapil scored a huge 175 runs off 138 balls against a crucial match against Zimbabwe during the 1983 World Cup. India won the match by 31 runs and went on to win its first World Cup Trophy, the other being the recent one earlier in 2011. The innings played by Kapil Dev is regarded as one of the Top 10 ODI Batting Performances of all times by the Wisden magazine.

Kapil Dev played 131 Test matches and played 225 ODI matches throughout his career. He served as the Coach of the Indian Cricket team from October 1999 to August 2000 but resigned after match fixing allegations were imposed upon him.

He was captain when India won the world cup in 1983. He was titled as the Indian Cricketer of the Century in 2002 by Wisden.

Trivia

He has won the prestigious **Arjuna Award**, the **Padma Shri** and the **Padma Bhushan**.

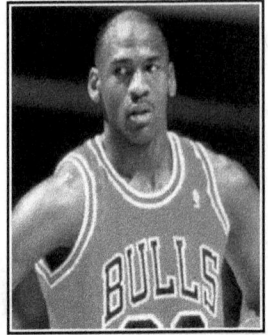

MICHAEL JORDAN

Michael Jeffrey Jordan is a former American professional basketball player. He was born in Brookyln, New York on February 17, 1963. As a kid, Michael Jordan was more interested in playing baseball rather than basketball but he soon started to play basketball to try and follow the footsteps of his elder brother, Larry, whom he idolised growing up.

He decided to enter the National Basketball Association (NBA) draft after winning the Naismith College Player of the Year Award in 1984.

Jordan's individual accomplishments include ten All-NBA First Team designations, five MVP awards, ten scoring titles, fourteen NBA All-Star Game appearances, nine All-Defensive First Team honors, three All-Star Game MVP awards, three steals titles, six NBA Finals MVP awards and the 1988 NBA Defensive Player of the Year Award.

In 1993, tragedy struck Jordan's seemingly perfect life. On July 23, 1993, his father James was murdered off Interstate 95 in North Carolina. Two locals had robbed him, shot him in the chest and threw his body in a swamp.

Three months later, in 1993, he announced his retirement. In 1994, he played baseball for Chicago White Sox, though the season didn't go that well.

He retired for good following the 2002-03 seasons and was subsequently dismissed as President of the Washington Wizards.

Trivia

His leaping ability, illustrated by performing slam dunks from the free throw line in slam dunk contests, earned him the nicknames, 'Air Jordan' and 'His Airness'.

Quote

"I've missed more than 9000 shots in my career. I've lost almost 300 games. 26 times. I've been trusted to take the game winning shot and missed. I've failed over and over and over again in my life. And that is why I succeed."

MUHAMMAD ALI

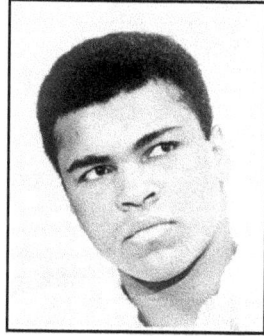

Born on January 17, 1942, Muhammad Ali is a former American professional boxer, a philanthropist and a social activist. Considered a cultural icon, Ali was both idolised and vilified

Originally known as Cassius Clay, Ali changed his name after joining the 'Nation of Islam' in 1964, subsequently converting to 'Sunni Islam' in 1975, and more recently to Sufism.

At the age of 12, Ali discovered his talent for boxing through an odd twist of fate.

In 1967, three years after Ali had won the 'World Heavyweight Championship', he was publicly vilified for his refusal to be conscripted into the US military. The decision, he said, was based on his religious beliefs.

Though Ali cleared his name after a lengthy court battle. The boxing association took away his title and also suspended him from the sport for three and a half years.

He came back in the ring in 1970 and knocked out Jerry Quarry in October in Atlanta. Ali fought the reigning heavyweight champion George Foreman in 1974 and became the heavyweight champion of the world.

In 1981, Ali fought his last bout, losing his heavyweight title to Trevor Berbick.

In his retirement, Ali has devoted much of his time to philanthropy.

Trivia

He opened the 'Muhammad Ali Centre' in his hometown, Louisville, in 2005. He also received the 'Presidential Medal of Freedom' from President George W. Bush.

PELÉ

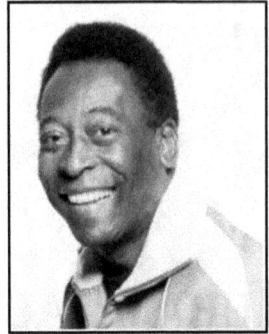

A lso known by the name of **The Black Pearl**, Pelé was born on October 23, 1940 in Tres Coracoes, Minas Gerais,Brazil.

Simply he was, and for many people still is, the greatest football player of the world. Not a single thing was impossible for him: he won *three* World Cups with his National Team of Brazil (Sweden 1958, Chile 1962, Mexico 1970).

He scored more than 1200 goals during his long career (more than 1300 official matches). He also won many national Leagues and Continental Cup ("Copa Libertadores"), with his team, the Santos Futebol Clube (of Brazilian 'São Paulo' State).

In the Sixties he was nicknamed "O Rei" (The King) and in the Seventies 95 people out of 100 knew his name. ("Wow, man, you're popular!" said Robert Redford, some years ago, after seeing Pelé give dozens of autographs in New York, while he was not asked for one). In the late, 1960's, when he and his team, Santos, went to Nigeria to play a few friendly matches, the ongoing civil war stopped for the duration of his visit.

He finished his career in the New York Cosmos, in 1977. Now he is a United Nation's Ambassador and has been also Minister for Sports in his country, but for the people who saw him make magics with his right foot, he is, now and forever, the greatest footballer in the world, and the one and only "King".

Trivia
He is the only player to have won *three* FIFA World Cup titles (1958, 1962, 1970).

Quote
"Enthusiasm is everything. It must be taut and vibrating like a guitar string."

📹 📹

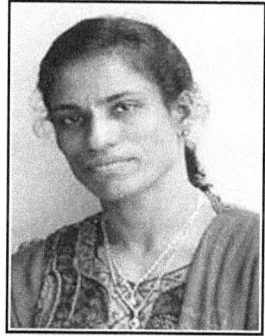

P.T. USHA

P.T. Usha was born on June 27, 1964. She is an Indian athlete from the state of Kerala. PT Usha has been associated with Indian athletics since 1979. She is regarded as one of the greatest athletes India has ever produced and is often called the 'Queen of Indian track and field'. She is nicknamed *Payyoli Express*. Currently she runs the 'Usha School of Athletics' at Koyilandy in Kerala.

P.T. Usha was born in the village of Payyoli, Kozhikode District, Kerala. In 1976, the Kerala State Government started a Sports School for women, and Usha was chosen to represent her district.

In the 10th Asian Games held at Seoul in 1986, PT Usha won four gold and one silver medals in the track and field events. Here she created new Asian Games records in all the events she participated.

She won five golds at the '6th Asian Track and Field Championship' at Jakarta in 1985. Her six medals at the same meet is a record for a single athlete in a single international meet. Usha has won 101 international medals so far. She is employed as an officer in the Southern Railways. In 1985, she was conferred the **Padma Shri** and the **Arjuna Award**.

Trivia

P.T. Usha's full name is Pilavullakandi Thekkeparambil Usha.

🎥 🎥

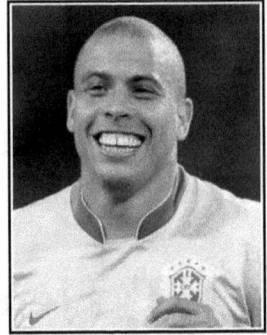

RONALDO

Commonly known as Ronaldo, Ronaldo Luís Nazário de Lima is a retired Brazilian footballer who last played for Corinthians.

Born on September 18, 1976, Ronaldo is widely considered to be the greatest 'pure' striker in the history of the modern game, and by some accounts, in the history of football.

He has been one of the most prolific scorers in the world in the late 1990s and the early 2000s. He won his first 'Ballon d'Or' (the Golden Ball) as the European Footballer of the Year in 1997 at the age of 21 and the second one at the age of 26.

Additionally, he and French footballer Zinedine Zidane are the only two men to have won the FIFA Player of the Year Award three times.

He was named as one of the best starting eleven of all time by France Football and was named to the FIFA 100 – a list of the greatest footballers compiled by fellow countryman Pelé – in 2007.

In 2010, he was voted goal.com's 'Player of the Decade' in an online poll, gathering 43.63 percent of all votes. On 23 February 2010, Ronaldo announced that he will retire after the 2011 season, signing a two-year contract extension with the Corinthians at the same time.

Trivia

Ronaldo has played for Brazil in 97 international matches, amassing 62 goals.

SACHIN TENDULKAR

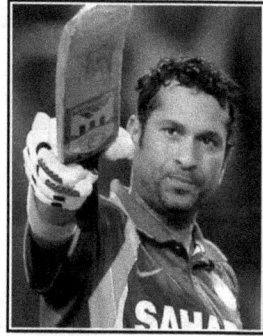

Sachin Ramesh Tendulkar also known as 'The God of Cricket' is regarded as one of the greatest batsmen in the history of cricket.

Tendulkar is the first and only player in Test Cricket to have scored 50 centuries and the first cricketer to score 100 centuries in all International Cricket combined. He holds the world record of 100 centuries (49 ODI & 51 Test Cricket) in international cricket.

Born into a Rajapur Saraswat Brahmin family in Bombay (now Mumbai), his father, Ramesh Tendulkar was a Marathi novelist. He was named 'Sachin' because his father was as great fan of the famous music director, Sachin Dev Burman. Tendulkar's elder brother, 'Ajit' encouraged him to play cricket. When he was young, Sachin would practise for hours in the nets.

At the age of 13, Tendulkar made his debut in club cricket for the Cricket Club of India. When he was just 15 years old, Sachin scored 100 not out in his debut first class match for Bomaby against Gujarat making him the youngest Indian to score a century on first-class debut. After the veteran player, Sunil Manohar Gavaskar, Sachin is the only cricketer to be nicknamed as the 'Little Master'. Sachin is married to a doctor named Anjali, who happens to be the daughter of a Gujarati industrialist.

This great cricketer has been awarded with innumerable honours and appreciations, across the globe. He has been conferrerd with **Padma Vibushan**, India's second highest civilian award in 2008. He is also the recipient of **Rajiv Gandhi Khel Ratna Award**, Indian highest honour given for achievement in sports. Besides this, he was awarded the 'BCCI Cricketer of the Year' award on May 31, 2011 after India won the prestigious World Cup.

Trivia

Sachin Ramesh Tendulkar went to Shradashram Vidyamandir in Mumbai, where he began his cricketing career under his coach, Ramakant Achrekar.

📹 📹

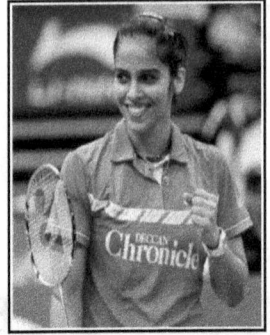

SAINA NEHWAL

Saina Nehwal was born on March 17, 1990. She is an Indian badminton player. Saina was born in Hyderabad, India to Dr. Harvir Singh and Usha Nehwal, both of whom were top badminton players in Haryana, India.

Saina has been the under 19 national champion. She has won the Asian Satellite Badminton tournament twice and is the first player to do so. She became the first Indian women to win a four-star tournament, the Philippines Open in 2006. In 2008, she became the first Indian women to win the World Junior Badminton Championship. She also became the first Indian woman to reach the quarter finals at the Olympic Games. In 2008, she won the Chinese Taipei Open. She was named the 'Most Promising Player' in 2008.

In 2009, she won the BWG Super series and the most prominent badminton series 'Indonesia Open'. She was awarded the **'Arjuna'** Award in 2009 and her coach Gopichand won the **'Dronacharya'** Award at the same time. Saina was also awarded the **Padma Shri** in 2010.

Saina has been awarded the highest national sporting award given to players, **Rajiv Gandhi Khel Ratna Award** in 2010. In the Commonwealth Games held in India, Sania won a gold medal for women's single's badminton event. In December 2010, Saina won the Hong Kong super series.

Saina Nehwal has been voted the third best badminton player of the year 2010 by Badzine, an international badminton magazine. She won the 2010 Indian Open Grand Prix gold. She was ranked world no 3 in women's single's badminton rankings and in July 2010 she reached the world ranking no 2.

Saina managed to win the 'Swiss Open Grand Prix' in March 2011. After that she hasn't managed a win in any of the championships she played in which were Indian Open Super Series, Malaysian Open Grand Prix Gold tournament, 2011 BWF Double Star Surdiman Cup, Thailand Open GP Gold, Singapore Open Super Series and Indonesian Open Super Series Premiere.

SUNIL GAVASKAR

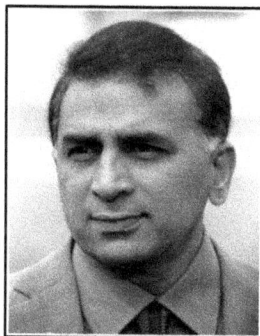

Born on July 10, 1949, Sunil Gavaskar is a former Indian batsman. His record of 34 Test centuries took 20 years to be broken by Sachin Tendulkar in 2005.

The record-setting batsman has been a national hero to cricket fans. His spectacular career began with a bang with scoring 774 runs against West Indies in 1971.

He was the first batsman to score 0,000 runs in Test Cricket.

He was the greatest Test scorer with the highest number of centuries to his credit during his times.

He has served as a captain of the Indian cricket team for a long time. However, the team did not fare well during his captaincy. He led the team in 47 Test matches, out of which, the team won nine, eight were lost and 30 were drawn.

Under his captaincy, the Indian team won 14 ODI matches, lost 21 and two went without any result out of the 37 ODI matches.

Gavaskar played his last Test match against Pakistan in March 1987 and scored 117 runs. His last ODI match was against England in November 1987 in which he scored just four runs.

He dominated the Indian cricket and became famous for his meticulous approach as well as his distinctive headgear.

He became a commentator and columnist after he retired in 1988.

Trivia

Sunil Manohar Gavaskar has been conferred with **Padma Bhushan**. He has written four books on cricket and an autobiography, titled 'Sunny days'. A Test Cricket Series between India and Australia has been jointly named after him and the Australian Cricketer, Allan Border as the 'Border-Gavaskar Trophy'.

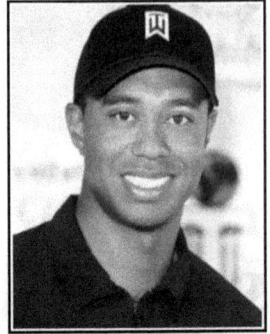

TIGER WOODS

Eldrick Tont 'Tiger' Woods was born on December 30, 1975. He is an American professional golfer whose achievements to date rank him among the most successful golfers of all time.

Formerly the World No 1, Tigre Woods is the highest-paid professional athlete in the world, having earned an estimated US$90.5 million from winnings and endorsements in 2010.

Woods has won 14 professional major golf championships, the second highest of any male player and 71 PGA Tour events. He is the third all time behind Sam Snead and Nicklaus.

He has more career PGA Tour wins and career major wins than any other active golfer. He is the youngest player to achieve the career Grand Slam and the youngest and fastest to win 50 tournaments on tour.

Woods is the second golfer, after Jack Nicklaus, to have achieved a career Grand Slam three times.

Woods has won 16 World Golf Championships. Additionally, he has won at least one of those events in each of the first 11 years after they began in 1999.

He married Elin Nordegren in 2004 and the couple had two children before they announced divorce in 2010. The media reports accused Woods of having an extra marital affair.

His multiple infidelities were revealed by over a dozen women, through many worldwide media sources.

He has been awarded **PGA Player of the Year**, a record **ten times**, the **Byron Nelson Award** for lowest adjusted scoring average a record about **eight times**.

Trivia

On December 11, 2009, Woods announced he would take an indefinite leave from professional golf to focus on his marriage after he admitted infidelity and returned to Golf on April 8, 2010.

🎥 🎥

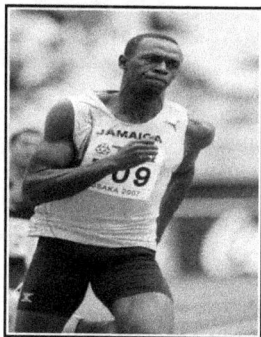

USAIN ST. LEO BOLT

Usain St. Leo Bolt, the Fastest Man on Earth born on August 21, 1986, is a Jamaican sprinter and a five-time World and three-time Olympic gold medallist. He is the world record and Olympic record holder in the 100 metres, the 200 metres and the 4×100 metres relay. He is the *reigning Olympic champion* in these three events.

Bolt won a 200 m gold medal at the 2002 World Junior Championships, making him the competition's youngest-ever gold medallist. In 2004, at the CARIFTA Games, he became the first junior sprinter to run the 200 m in under 20 seconds with a time of 19.93 s, breaking the previous world junior record held by Roy Martin by two-tenths of a second. He turned professional in 2004, and although he competed at the 2004 Summer Olympics, he missed most of the next two seasons due to injuries. In 2007, he broke Don Quarrie's 200 m Jamaican record with a run of 19.75 s.

His 2008 season began with his first world record performance – a 100 m world record of 9.72 s – and culminated in world and Olympic records in both the 100 m and 200 m events at the 2008 Beijing Summer Olympics. He ran 9.69 s for the 100 m and 19.30 s in the 200 m, and also set a 4×100 m relay record of 37.10 s with the Jamaican team.

Trivia

His 2009 record breaking margin over 100 m is the highest since the start of digital time measurements. His achievements in sprinting have earned him the media nickname, "Lightning Bolt", and awards including the IAAF World Athlete of the Year, Track & Field Athlete of the Year, and Laureus Sportsman of the Year.

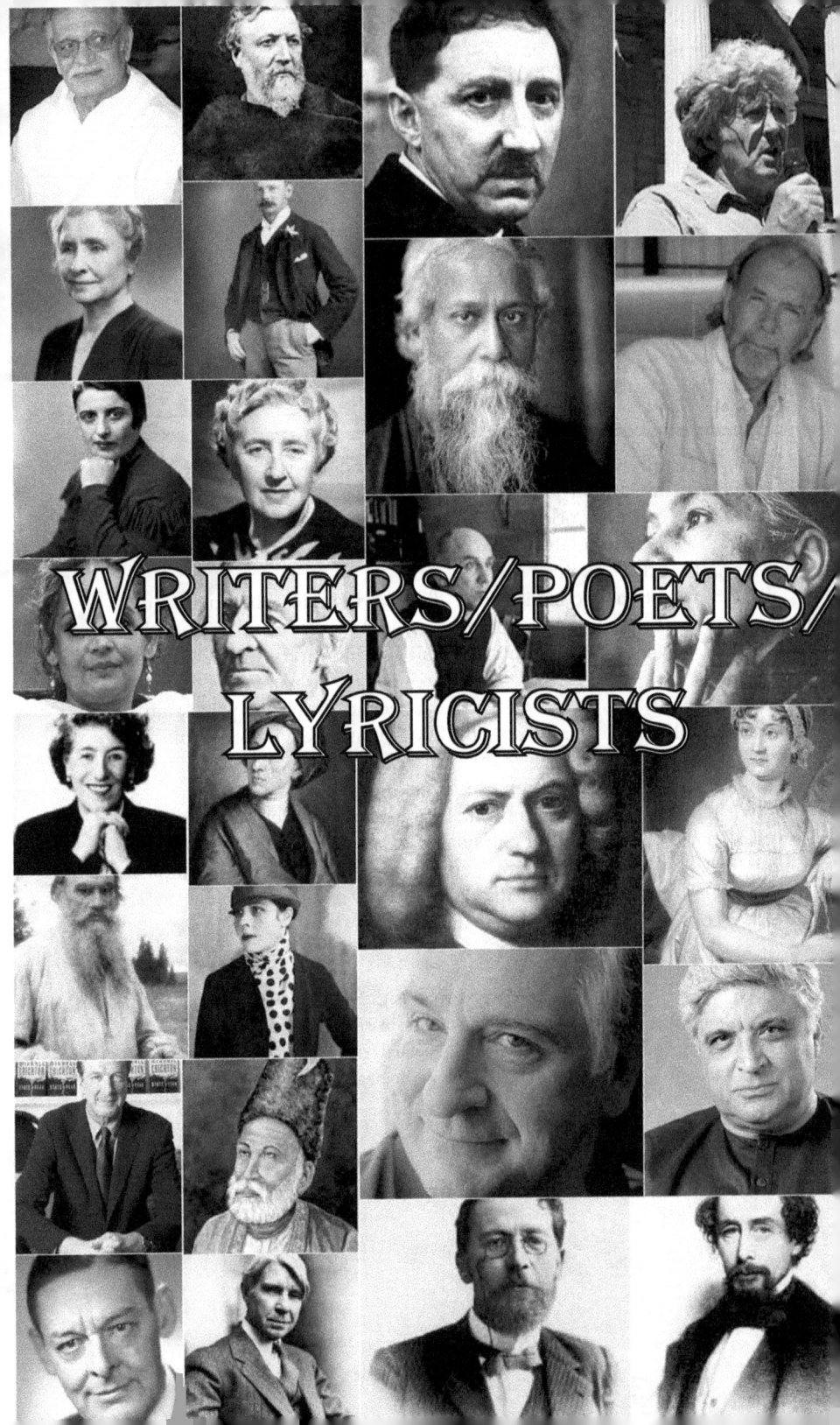

WRITERS/POETS/ LYRICISTS

AGATHA CHRISTIE

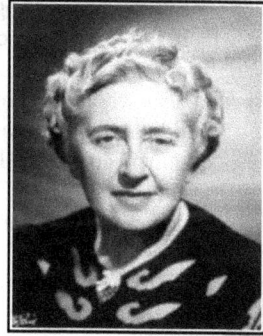

Dame Agatha Christie was born on September 15, 1890. She was a British crime writer of novels, short stories and plays. She also wrote romances under the name, Mary Westmacott.

Agatha Chritsie was born in Torquay, Devon, England. While she never received any formal schooling, she did not lack an education. Her father taught her mathematics via story problems, and the family played question-and-answer games. Agatha made up stories from a very early age and invented a number of imaginary friends and paracosms.

During the First World War, she worked at a hospital as a nurse. She later worked at a hospital pharmacy, a job that influenced her work, as many of the murders in her books are carried out with poison.

Despite a turbulent courtship, on Christmas Eve 1914, Agatha married Archibald Christie, an aviator in the Royal Flying Corps. The couple had one daughter, Rosalind Hicks. The Christies divorced in 1928. In 1930, Christie married an archaeologist. Their marriage was especially happy in the early years and remained so until Christie's death in 1976.

Agatha Christie's first novel, *The Mysterious Affair at Styles* was published in 1920 and introduced the long-running character detective, Hercule Poirot appeared in 33 of Christie's novels and 54 short stories. Her other well-known character, Miss Marple, was introduced in *The Tuesday Night Club* in 1927 (short story) and was based on women like Christie's grandmother and her cronies.

Christie wrote two novels, *Curtain*, and *Sleeping Murder*, intended as the last cases of these two great detectives, Hercule Poirot and Jane Marple. Both books were sealed in a bank vault for over thirty years and were released for publication by Christie only at the end of her life. These publications came on the heels of the success of the film version of *Murder on the Orient Express* in 1974.

Agatha Christie was revered as a **master of suspense**, plotting, and characterisation by most of her contemporaries.

Christie has been portrayed on a number of occasions in film and television. Several biographical programs have been made, such as the

2004 BBC television programme entitled *Agatha Christie: A Life in Pictures*, in which she is portrayed by Olivia Williams, Anna Massey, and Bonnie Wright. Christie has also been parodied on screen, such as in the film, *Murder by Indecision*, which featured the character, "Agatha Crispy".

In 2004, the Japanese broadcasting company Nippon Hōsō Kyōkai turned Poirot and Marple into animated characters in the anime series, Agatha Christie's Great Detectives Poirot and Marple, introducing Mabel West and her duck Oliver as new characters.

Agatha Christie died on January 12, 1976.

Trivia

At one point in her successful career, Agatha Christie actually owned eight different houses. Many of these were used as the houses in many of her novels, such as: Taken at the Flood, Dead Man's Folly, Five Little Pigs, Crooked House, etc.

Quote

"Crime is terribly revealing. Try and vary your methods as you will, your tastes, your habits, your atitude of mind and your soul is revealed by your actions."

CHARLES DICKENS

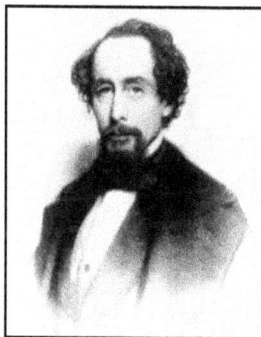

Charles John Huffam Dickens, usually called Charles Dickens, was born on February 7, 1812. He was an English novelist, the greatest of the Victorian period.

Charles was bon to John and Elizabeth Dickens. His father used to work as a clerk in the Navy-Pay office. Having a poor head for finances, he found himself imprisoned for debt in 1824. His wife and children, except Charles, joined him in the Marshalsea Prison. Charles was put to work at Warren's Blacking Factory.

He attended a school in London from 1824 to 1827. He later became a reporter and started writing for a newspaper.

Many of his writings were originally published serially, in monthly instalments or parts. Dickens often created the episodes as they were being serialised. This practice kept the public looking forward to the next instalment.

The first series of *Sketches by Boz* was published in 1836. Later, Dickens was hired to write short texts to accompany a series of humorous sporting illustrations by a popular artist, *Robert Seymour*.

Then, Dickens altered the initial conception of *The Pickwick Papers*, which became a novel and was a huge success. After its success, he embarked on a full-time career as novelist.

Some of his other works include *Master Humphrey's Clock, The Old Curiosity Shop, The Chimes, The Cricket* and the *Hearth*.

Dickens' work has been highly praised for its realism, comedy and mastery of prose, unique personalities and concern for social reform by famous writers.

He suffered a mild stroke in 1869 and another on June 8, 1870. He died on June 9, 1870.

Trivia

Dickens enjoyed a wider popularity and fame than any previous author during his lifetime.

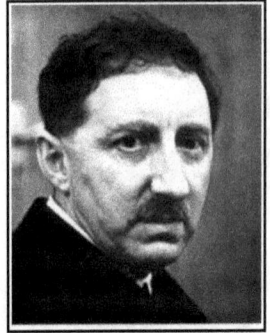

E.M. FORSTER

Edward Morgan Forster (January 1, 1879 – June 7, 1970) was an English novelist, short story writer, essayist and a liberalist.

Best known for his ironic and well-plotted novels examining class difference, Forster's humanistic impulse towards understanding and sympathy may be aptly summed up in the epigraph to his 1910 novel, *Howards End: 'Only connect'*.

After having attended the Tonbridge School in Kent, Forster went to King's College, Cambridge between 1897 and 1901. After leaving the University, he visited Egypt, Germany and India with the classicist Goldsworthy Lowes Dickinson in 1914.

He had five novels published in his lifetime. His first novel was *Where Angels Fear to Tread* (1905), *The Longest Journey* (1907), *A Room with a View* (1908), *Howards End* (1910), *A Passage to India* (1924).

He was in India in the early 1920s and *The Hill of Devi* is his non-fictional account of the trip. After returning from India, he completed his last novel, *A Passage to India* in 1924, for which he won the **James Tait Black Memorial Prize** for fiction.

Forster became a successful broadcaster on the BBC Radio in the 1930s and 1940s.

Forster is noted for his use of symbolism as a technique in his novels. He has been criticised for his attachment to mysticism. One example of his symbolism is the 'wych elm tree' in *Howards End* and 'Mrs Moore' in *A Passage to India* has a mystical link with the past and a striking ability to connect with people from beyond their own circles.

Trivia

His name was officially registered as Henry Morgan Forster but at his baptism, he was accidentally named Edward Morgan Forster.

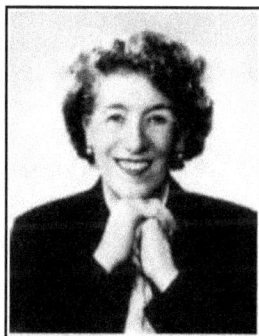

ENID BLYTON

Enid Blyton (August 11, 1897 – November 28, 1968) was an English children's writer also known as 'Mary Pollock'.

She was noted for numerous series of books based on recurring characters and designed for different age groups. Her books have enjoyed huge success in many parts of the world, and have sold over 600 million copies.

One of the most widely known characters is *Noddy*, intended for early years readers. Her main work is the genre of young readers' novels in which children have their own adventures with minimal adult help.

Series of such books by her include – *The Famous Five* (21 novels, 1942–1963), the *Five Find-Outers and Dog*, (15 novels, 1943–1961) as well as *The Secret Seven* (15 novels, 1949–1963).

Enid announced her marriage to Hugh Alexander Pollock, who was the editor of the book department in the publishing firm of George Newnes in 1924. The couple had two children.

Her work basically involved children's adventure stories and fantasy and sometimes, magic. Her books were and still are enormously popular throughout the Commonwealth – as translations in the former Yugoslavia, Japan; as adaptations in Arabic; and across most of the globe. Her work has been translated into nearly *90 languages*.

She has an estimated **800 books** to her credit over roughly 40 years. 'Chorion Limited of London' now owns and handles the intellectual properties and character brands of *Blyton's Noddy* and the well-known series of the *Famous Five*.

Trivia

As a child, Enid Blyton faced some medical problems that brought her very close to death.

GULZAR

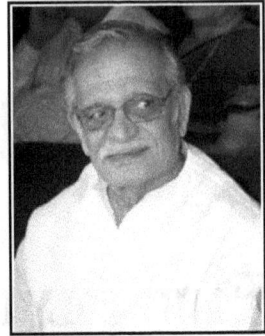

Sampooran Singh Kalra was born on August 18, 1936. Popularly known by his pen name Gulzar, he is an Indian poet, lyricist and director. He primarily writes in Hindi-Urdu and has also written in Punjabi including several dialects of Hindi, such as *Braj Bhasha, Khariboli, Haryanvi* and *Marwari*.

Gulzar was awarded the 'Padma Bhushan' in 2004 for his contribution to the arts and the 'Sahitya Akademi Award' in 2002.

In 2009, he won the 'Academy Award' for the Best Original Song for 'Jai Ho' in the film, *Slumdog Millionaire* (2008). On January 31, 2010, the same song won him a **Grammy Award** in the category of Grammy Award for Best Song Written for a Motion Picture, Television or Other Visual Media.

Gulzar's poetry is partly published in three compilations: *Chand Pukhraaj Ka, Raat Pashminey Ki* and *Pandrah Paanch Pachattar* (15-05-75). His short stories are published in *Raavi-paar* (Dustkhat in Pakistan) and 'Dhuan'.

As a lyricist, Gulzar is best known for his association with the music directors, Rahul Dev Burman, A. R. Rahman and Vishal Bhardwaj. He has also worked with other leading Bollywood music directors including Sachin Dev Burman, Salil Chowdhury, Hemant Kumar, Madan Mohan and Shankar–Ehsaan–Loy.

Trivia

His biography is written by his daughter, Meghna Gulzar.

Quote

"Music has a natural place in our lives. Music fills our spaces naturally. It will always be dear to us."

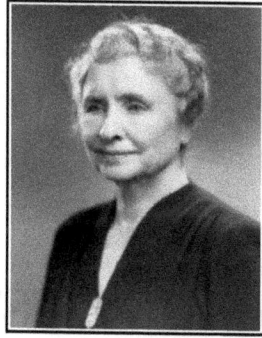

HELEN KELLER

An author, political activist and lecturer, Helen Keller was the first deaf and blind person to be a graduate. Her life is an example of how perseverance can overcome obstacles.

Helen Keller was born on June 27, 1880 in Tuscumbia, Alabama.

When she was one year and seven months old, she suffered from fever, assumed to be scarlet fever that left her deaf and blind. She was recommended to the Perkins Institute for the Blind in Boston by Alexander Graham Bell.

She met her teacher, Anne Sullivan in the Perkins Institute. Sullivan discovered a unique way to teach Helen words and their meanings. She once held Helen's hand under the flowing water. As the water fell on her hand, Sullivan wrote the alphabets of the word, 'water' one by one on her arm. Helen tried to grasp every motion felt on her arm and realised that the substance falling on her hand was called 'water'.

Sullivan's teaching abilities and Helen's will to learn helped her to pass examinations, learn five languages and write twelve books, including her autobiography, 'The Story of My Life'.

She was involved in campaigns for women's rights at her college level, which laid the foundation for her as a socialist. Helen also wrote articles for 'The Masses', a socialist journal. She devoted her life and travelled around the world to raise funds for the *American Foundation of the Blind*.

Helen Keller died in Westport, Connecticut, on June 1, 1968.

Trivia

Helen had a protruding left eye, due to which she was usually photographed in profile. Both her eyes were later replaced with glass eyes for 'medical and cosmetic' reasons.

Quote

"I can see, and that is why I can be happy, in what you call the dark, but which to me is golden. I can see a God-made world, not a man-made world."

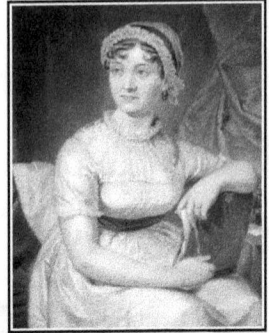

JANE AUSTEN

Jane Austen (December 16, 1775 – July 18, 1817) was an English novelist whose works of romantic fiction, set among the landed gentry, earned her a place as one of the most widely read writers in English literature, her realism and biting social commentary cementing her historical importance among scholars and critics.

She was educated primarily by her father and elder brothers as well as through her own reading. The steadfast support of her family was critical to her development as a professional writer.

Her artistic apprenticeship lasted from her teenage years, until she was about 35 years old. During this period, she experimented with various literary forms, including the epistolary novel which she tried, then abandoned and wrote, and extensively revised three major novels. She also began a fourth one.

From 1811 until 1816, many of her books were released including *Sense and Sensibility* (1811), *Pride and Prejudice* (1813), *Mansfield Park* (1814) and *Emma* (1816), she achieved success as a great writer.

She wrote two additional novels, *Northanger Abbey* and *Persuasion*, both published posthumously in 1818, and began a third, which was eventually titled *Sanditon*, but died before completing it.

Trivia

Biographical information concerning Jane Austen is 'famously scarce', according to one biographer. Only some personal and family letters remain as her sister, Cassandra, burnt 'the greater part' of the ones she kept and censored those she did not destroy.

JAVED AKHTAR

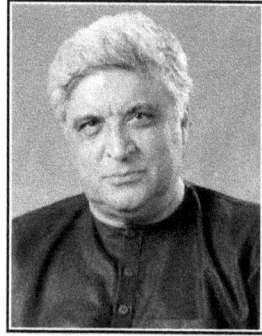

Javed Akhtar was born on January 17, 1945 in Gwalior. He is a poet, lyricist and scriptwriter from India. Some of his most successful work was done in the late 1970s and 1980s with Salim Khan. The script-writing duo Salim-Javed is credited with many good and long-lasting songs. Both of them delivered some beautiful hits like *Zanjeer, Deewar, Haathi Mere Saathi, Don* and many more.

Javed Akhtar continues to be a prominent figure in Bollywood and is one of the most popular lyricists in the industry. His original name was Jadoo, taken from a line in a poem written by his father – 'Lamha, lamha kisi jadoo ka fasana hoga'. He was given an official name of Javed

Javed Akhtar has also won about seven 'Filmfare' awards. He has been conferred with **Padma Shri** and **Padma Bhushan**.

A multi-talented personality, Javed Akhtar continues to get rave reviews and awards for his works. His first collection of Urdu poems was released in the year, 1995. It was also released as an album and sold many CDs.

The famous artist, M.F. Hussain is said to have painted around 16 canvases inspired from Javed Akhtar's poems.

He not only excels as a poet but also as a scriptwriter and lyricist.

Trivia

After the success of 'Don', it was remade in Tamil as 'Billa' starring Rajinikanth, but the story writers were the same, Salim-Javed, in it and they made a few changes in the script, here and there.

Quote

"We put women on a pedestal. So we do not consider them to be human beings."

JEROME KLAPKA JEROME

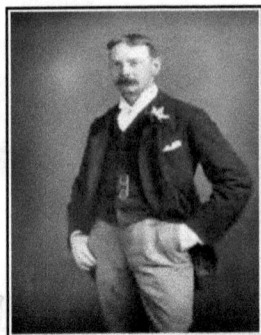

J erome Klapka Jerome (May 2, 1859 – June 14, 1927) was an English writer and humorist, best known for the humorous travelogue, *Three Men in a Boat*.

Jerome was born in Caldmore, Walsall, England, and was brought up in poverty in London. He attended St Marylebone Grammar School.

Jerome was the fourth child of Jerome Clapp, an iron monger and lay preacher who dabbled in architecture, and Marguerite Jones. Jerome K Jerome was registered, like his father's amended name, as Jerome Clapp Jerome, and the Klapka appears to be a later variation.

Owing to bad investments in the local mining industry, the family suffered poverty, and debt collectors often visited. This was an experience of Jerome's life, which he has described vividly in his autobiography, *My Life and Times.*

His other works include the essay collections, 'Idle Thoughts of an Idle Fellow' and 'Second Thoughts of an Idle Fellow'. Several other novels are credited in his name including *Three Men on the Bummel* is a sequel to *Three Men in a Boat.*

Trivia

The young Jerome wished to go into politics or be a man of letters but the death of his father at the age of 13 and his mother at the age of 15, forced him to quit his studies and find work to support himself. He was employed at the London and North-Western Railway, initially collecting coal that fell along the railway, remaining there for about four years.

JONATHAN SWIFT

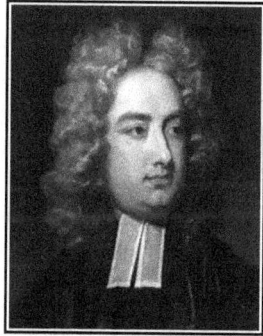

Jonathan Swift (November 30, 1667 – October 19, 1745) was an Anglo-Irish satirist, political pamphleteer, essayist and poet. Born in Dublin, Ireland, Swift began his education at the age of six. Later, he graduated from the Trinity College in 1686.

After the political turmoil during the Glorious Revolution, Swift came to England and became secretary to Sir William Temple, a diplomat and man of letters.

It was the period between 1696 and 1699 that Swift composed most of his first great work – *A Tale of a Tub*, a prose satire on the religious extremes represented by Roman Catholicism and Calvinism and *The Battle of the Books* in 1697. In 1699, Swift travelled to Ireland as chaplain and secretary to the Earl of Berkeley.

He is remembered for works, such as *Gulliver's Travels, A Journal to Stella, A Modest Proposal, Drapier's Letters, The Battle of the Books* and *An Argument Against Abolishing Christianity*.

Swift originally published all of his works under pseudonyms – such as Lemuel Gulliver, Isaac Bickerstaff, MB Drapier – or anonymously. He is also known for being a master of two styles of satire – the 'Horatian' and the 'Juvenalian styles'.

Swift's final trip to England took place in 1727. He published five volumes of 'Swift-Pope Miscellanies' between 1727 and 1736. Swift's ghastly 'A Beautiful Young Nymph Going to Bed' was published in 1731.

By 1735, his Meniere's disease became more acute, resulting in periods of dizziness and nausea.

After a prolonged illness, Swift died on October 19, 1745.

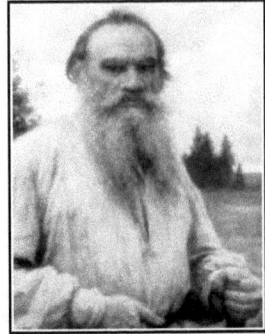

LEO TOLSTOY

Lev Nikolayevich Tolstoy (September 9, 1828 – November 20, 1910) was a Russian writer. He primarily wrote novels and short stories. Later in life, he also wrote plays and essays. Two of his most famous works – the novels, *War and Peace* and *Anna Karenina* – are acknowledged as a pinnacle of realistic fiction

Leo Tolstoy studied languages and law at the Kazan University for three years. Being dissatisfied with the school, he left Kazan without a degree, returned to his estate and educated himself independently.

Considered to be one of the world's greatest novelists, Tolstoy is equally known for his complicated persona and for his extreme moralistic views, which he adopted after a moral crisis and spiritual awakening in the 1870s. After this period, he also became noted as a moral thinker and social reformer.

His literal interpretation of the ethical teachings of Jesus caused him, in later life, to become a fervent Christian anarchist. His ideas on non-violent resistance are expressed in works, such as *The Kingdom of God Is Within You*. They had a profound impact on pivotal twentieth-century figures, such as Mahatma Gandhi and Martin Luther King, Jr.

He died of pneumonia at the age of 82.

Trivia

He was probably the first writer to have groupies. Towards the end of his life, there were nearly one hundred fans living in and around his home so that they could experience his greatness firsthand.

Quote

"Love is life. All, everything that I understand, I understand only because I love. Everything is, everything exists, only because I love. Everything is united by it alone. Love is God, and to die means that I, a particle of love, shall return to the general and eternal source."

MIRZA GHALIB

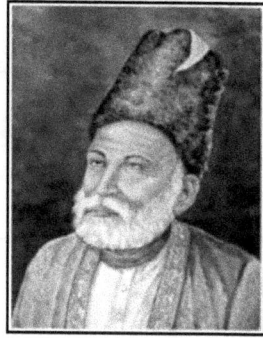

One of the best-known Urdu poets of all times, Mirza Ghalib is a name synonymous with Urdu poetry. Popularly known as Ghalib, Mirza Asadullah Baig Khan was born on December 27, 1796.

He wrote several 'ghazals' during his lifetime, which have since been interpreted and sung in many different ways.

Born in Agra, his father died in a battle when Ghalib was five years old. He was, then, looked after by his uncle, who also died when Ghalib was ten years old.

The death of his father and uncle during his early youth left Ghalib with no male-dominant figures. e then moved to Delhi.

There are no known records of Ghalib's formal education, although it was known that friends in Delhi were some of the most intelligent minds of the time.

He was married into a family of nobles, at the age of thirteen around 1810. He had seven children, none of whom survived.

Ghalib's fame came to him posthumously. He had himself had said during his lifetime that though his age ignored his greatness, his work would be recognised by later generations.

He also is arguably the most 'written about' among the Urdu poets.

The first complete English translation of Ghalib's love poems (ghazals) was written by Dr. Sarfaraz K Niazi, titled 'Love Sonnets of Ghalib', which was published in India and Pakistan.

Ghalib died in Delhi on February 15, 1869.

Trivia

Ghalib never worked as such for his livelihood and lived on state patronage, credit or generosity of his friends.

RABINDRANATH TAGORE

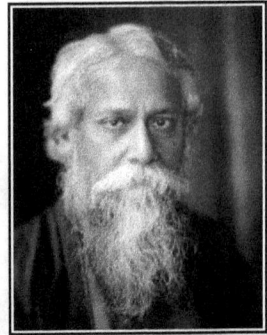

Rabindranath Tagore was born in the Jorasanko mansion in Calcutta (Kolkata) on May 7, 1861 to Debendranath Tagore and Sarada Devi.

Author of *Gitanjali* and its 'profoundly sensitive, fresh and beautiful verse', he became the first non-European Nobel laureate by earning the 1913 Nobel Prize in Literature. In translation, his poetry was viewed as spiritual and mercurial; his seemingly mesmeric persona, floccose locks, and empyreal garb garnered him a prophet-like aura in the West.

His 'elegant prose and magical poetry' remain largely unknown outside Bengal.

As a humanist, universalist, internationalist and strident anti-nationalist, he denounced the Raj and advocated for independence from Britain.

As an exponent of the Bengal Renaissance, he advanced a vast canon that comprised paintings, sketches and doodles, hundreds of texts, and some two thousand songs; his legacy endures also in the institution he founded, the Visva-Bharati University.

He started writing poetry at an age of 8. At the age of 16, he cheekily released his first substantial poems under the pseudonym, *Bhanusingha* (Sun Lion), his novels, stories, songs, dance-dramas, and essays spoke to topics – political and personal.

Gitanjali (Song Offerings), *Gora* (Fair-Faced), and *Ghare-Baire* (The Home and the World) are his best-known works, and his verse, short stories and novels were acclaimed for their lyricism, colloquialism, naturalism and unnatural contemplation. He penned two national anthems: the Republic of India's 'Jana Gana Mana' and Bangladesh's 'Amar Shonar Bangla'.

Trivia

He established the Bolpur Bramhacharya Ashram at Shantiniketan, a school based on the pattern of old Indian Ashram.

Quote

"I slept and dreamt that life was joy. I awoke and saw that life was service. I acted and behold, service was joy."

Ralph Waldo Emerson

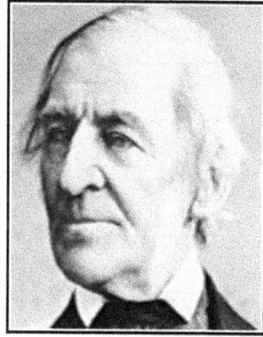

Ralph Waldo Emerson (May 25, 1803 – April 27, 1882) was an American essayist, lecturer and poet. He led the Transcendentalist Movement of the mid-19th century.

He was seen as a champion of individualism and a prescient critic of the countervailing pressures of the society. He disseminated his thoughts through dozens of published essays and more than 1,500 public lectures across the United States.

In his 1836 essay, *Nature*, Emerson formulated and expressed the philosophy of Transcendentalism, gradually moving away from the religious and social beliefs of his contemporaries.

Following this ground-breaking work, he gave a speech titled, *The American Scholar* in 1837, which Oliver Wendell Holmes Sr. considered to be America's 'Intellectual Declaration of Independence'.

Emerson's first two collections of essays – Essays: First Series and Essays: Second Series were published respectively in 1841 and 1844. They represent the core of his thinking, and include well-known essays, such as *The Over-Soul, Self-Reliance, The Poet, Circles* and the *Experience*.

Emerson wrote on a number of subjects, developing certain ideas such as freedom, individuality, the ability for humankind to realise almost anything and the relationship between the soul and the surrounding world. Emerson's 'Nature' was more philosophical than naturalistic, 'Philosophically considered, the universe is composed of Nature and the Soul'.

Trivia

Emerson's essays remain among the linchpins of American thinking and his work has greatly influenced the thinkers, writers and poets that have followed him.

ROBERT BROWNING

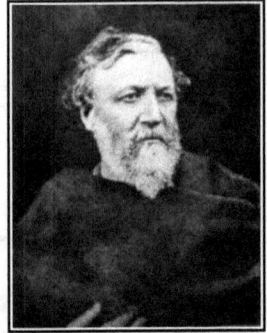

Robert Browning was born on May 7, 1812 in Camberwell, London. He was an English poet and playwright. His mastery of dramatic verse, especially dramatic monologues made him one of the foremost Victorian poets.

Browning was an extremely bright child and a voracious reader. He learned Greek, Latin, French and Italian by the time he was fourteen years old. He attended the University of London in 1828. In the 1830s, he tried to write verse drama for stage several times and realised that his talent lies in taking a single character.

He started writing poems during the same time. Some of his earlier works were *Paracelsus* (1835) and *Sordello* (1840).

He met the poet, Elizabeth Barrett in 1845. Although she was an invalid and very much under the control of a domineering father, they got married in 1846 and later eloped to Italy.

Barrett had been a more popular poet than Browning during their lifetimes. Some of his other works include *Collected Poems* (1862) and *Dramatis Personae* (1863). *The Ring and the Book* (1868-9), based on an 'old yellow book', which told of a Roman murder and trial, finally won him popularit .

The late 1860s were the peak of his career. Browning's influence continued to grow and finally led to the founding of the *Browning Society* in 1881. He died in 1889, on the same day when his final volume of verse, *Asolando*, was published.

Trivia

Elizabeth Barrett's love for Browning was demonstrated in the 'Sonnets from the Portuguese', and to her, he dedicated 'Men and Women' that contains his best poetry.

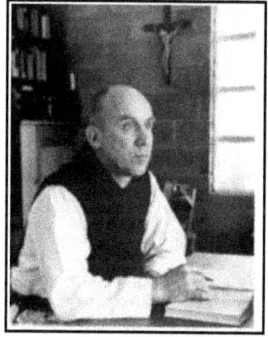

THOMAS MERTON

Thomas Merton was born on January 31, 1915 in Prades, Pyrénées-Orientales, France, to Owen Merton, a New Zealand painter, active in Europe and the United States, and Ruth Jenkins, an American Quaker and artist.

He was basically an Anglo-American Catholic **writer and mystic**. A Trappist monk of the Abbey of Gethsemani, he was a poet, a social activist and a student of comparative religion. He came to be known as Father Louis after he was ordained to the priesthood in 1949.

Thomas Merton wrote over 70 books, mostly on social justice spirituality, and a quiet pacifism, as well as scores of essays and reviews. His best-selling autobiography, *The Seven Storey Mountain*, sent scores of disillusioned World War II veterans, students, and even teenagers assembling at monasteries across the United States.

His autobiography was also featured in *National Review's* list of the 100 best non-fiction books of the centur .

Merton was a keen proponent of interfaith understanding. He pioneered dialogue with prominent Asian spiritual figures, including the Japanese writer, DT Suzuki, the Dalai Lama and the Vietnamese monk, Thich Nhat Hanh.

He was baptised in the Church of England, in accordance with his father's wishes. However, his father was often absent during Merton's upbringing.

Merton died in an accident on December 10, 1968, when he reached out to an electric fan while taking bath and was accidently electrocuted.

Trivia

Merton's influence has grown since his death and he is widely recognised as an important 20th-century Catholic mystic and thinker.

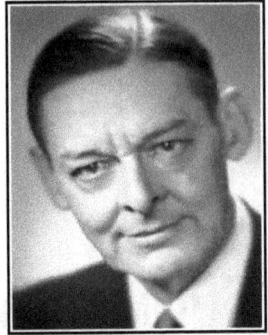

TS ELIOT

Tho**mas** Stearns, 'T S' Eliot (September 26, 1888 – January 4, 1965) was a playwright, literary critic and the most important English-language poet of the 20th century.

The poem that brought him fame was *The Love Song of J Alfred Prufrock*. Regarded as a masterpiece of the modernist movement, he started writing the poem in 1910 and it was published in Chicago in 1915.

This was followed with what have become some of the best-known poems in the English language, including *Gerontion*, *The Waste Land*, *The Hollow Men*, *Ash Wednesday*, and *Four Quartets*.

He is also known for his seven plays, the most important being *Murder in the Cathedral*.

He was awarded the **Nobel Prize in Literature** in 1948.

Eliot died of emphysema in London on January 4, 1965 after prolonged illness due to his heavy smoking. In accordance with Eliot's wishes, his ashes were taken to St Michael's Church in East Coker, the village from which his ancestors had emigrated to America.

Trivia

Although he was born an American, he moved to The United Kingdom in 1914 at the age of 25 and was naturalised as a British subject in 1927 at the age of 39.

www.ingramcontent.com/pod-product-compliance
Lightning Source LLC
Chambersburg PA
CBHW052037270326
41931CB00012B/2530